MEDICAL LIBRARY
ASSOCIATION *Guides*

DISCARD

Answering Consumer Health Questions

The Medical Library Association Guide for Reference Librarians

MICHELE SPATZ

NEAL-SCHUMAN PUBLISHERS, INC.
NEW YORK   LONDON

Published by Neal-Schuman Publishers, Inc.
100 William St., Suite 2004
New York, NY 10038

Printed and bound in the United States of America

The paper used in this publication meets the minimum requirements of American National Standard for Information Sciences—Permanence of Paper for Printed Library Materials, ANSI Z39.48-1992.

Library of Congress Cataloging-in-Publication Data

Spatz, Michele, 1954–
    Answering consumer health questions : the Medical Library Association guide for reference librarians / Michele Spatz.
        p. cm.
    Includes bibliographical references and index.
    ISBN 978-1-55570-632-6 (alk. paper)
    1. Medical libraries—Reference services—United States. 2. Health education—United States. 3. Consumer education—United States. I. Medical Library Association. II. Title.

Z675.M4S63 2008
025.5'27661—dc22
                                                            2008025035

Contents

List of Exhibits and Appendices

EXHIBITS

APPENDICES

Preface

Answering Consumer Health Questions: The Medical Library Association Guide for Reference Librarians is designed to help librarians provide health and medical information to their users. It is geared especially toward librarians who do not provide this type of information on a day-to-day basis, although even new and experienced medical librarians will find much here to use in their practice.

During every reference transaction, librarians serve as a bridge between a user with an information need and information resources that meet that need. However, when we provide consumer health and medical information, this bridge also includes a personal, more intimate dimension. Our role is not only to be informative, but also to provide tangible support to individuals who are seeking health information often because they are facing a personal dilemma, sometimes even a crisis, if not for themselves, then for others close to them.

In the realm of medical and health information, the librarian's role is to provide useful and appropriate resources that will help the patron understand a disease or condition and/or decide among various treatments. Happily, another role is to provide information that will help consumers learn what they can do to live longer, healthier lives. Perhaps in no other reference situation must librarians so carefully consider the personal and emotional impact knowledge can have on patrons. They must be in tune with an individual's fears, uncertainties, and desire for resolution and hope. In addition to possessing the skills needed to provide the appropriate informational resource, librarians must have an understanding of the psychology of health and medical consumers. Knowledge of psychology will help librarians make consumers feel secure enough to talk honestly about their concerns and needs. It will enable librarians to foresee the likely impact the information they provide will have on consumers and will enable them to help consumers deal with unpleasant and sometimes frightening information. Knowledge of psychology is also needed to help librarians deal with a diverse clientele—including challenging patrons—and to cope with the stress inherent in health- and medical-related reference work.

To a great extent, the open exchange of health and medical information and knowledge is a relatively recent development. Until the latter part of the twentieth century, medical knowledge was not intended for public consumption. It was deemed too complex and too inaccessible and thus beyond the layperson's understanding. It was closed off from the public domain, the preserve of a select few. For centuries, the practice of medicine had entwined men and magic to shape our early perceptions of who should have access to knowledge so closely linked with life and with death itself. It was rooted in secrecy and inspired fear and awe.

By providing the most useful information in an empathetic manner, librarians bridge the practical and the emotional. Requests for health information are often wrapped in feelings—fear, anxiety, sadness, helplessness, anger, frustration, and sometimes even joy. Librarians today must couple appropriate information-retrieval skills with knowledge of human behavior in order to meet people's health information needs. Librarians need to remember the roots of secrecy from which modern medicine has grown, appreciate the deeply individual impact of health conditions and diagnoses on the consumer, and respond appropriately, knowledgeably, and compassionately.

Key Features

The author has strived to produce a book that is both accessible and practical. Medical jargon is excluded, and terms are explained in layperson's language.

Italicized vignettes are interspersed throughout the text, providing scenarios that illustrate the concepts discussed in the narration.

Exhibits provide a multitude of information and advice, including:

- tips on numerous topics,

- recommended resources, and

- templates (e.g., financial toolkit; health information request; sample disclaimers; rules of conduct; unacceptable behavior incident report; sample patron complaint policy; stress mapper; reducing stress worksheet).

Organization

Answering Consumer Health Questions explores reference interaction from a behavioral perspective and offers appropriate approaches for responding to individuals in a wide variety of circumstances. The chapters address the most pressing issues librarians face in offering health information to consumers.

Chapter 1, "Professional Practice: Understanding and Reaching Out to the Health Information Seeker," discusses the unique aspects of this type of reference work, the common emotions and concerns of consumers seeking medical and health information, and appropriate responses on the part of librarians. Also discussed is the importance of promotion and outreach in getting the word out that the library is a trusted place to turn to for health and medical information.

Chapter 2, "Professional Interactions: Communication Guidelines and Strategies," focuses on the importance of nonverbal and verbal communication and on the strategies that can be used to maximize communication with consumers; it provides advice on how to handle unpleasant news and explains the importance of "compassionate neutrality"; and it offers guidelines for e-mail, virtual reference, and telephone reference.

Chapter 3, "Professional Ethics of Providing Health Information," explores moral and religious conflicts; personal feelings, emotions, and opinions; privacy and confidentiality; and ethics involved in service to special audiences. Included at the end of the chapter are the Medical Library Association Code of Ethics for Health Sciences Librarianship, the American Library Association's Code of Ethics, and the American Library Association's Library Bill of Rights.

Chapter 4, "Legal Issues in Health Information Delivery," reviews potential legal issues, including practicing medicine without a license, defamation of character, the constitutional right to know, and safeguards for professional practice. The chapter also offers tips for clear communication.

Chapter 5, "Serving the Health Information Needs of Diverse Individuals," addresses the needs of our diverse clientele, including the disabled; children and youth; patrons with mental health disorders; minority and culturally diverse individuals; and lesbian, gay, bisexual, and transgender individuals.

Chapter 6, "The Difficult Patron," offers tips for interacting with the most challenging patrons.

The final chapter, "Self-care for the Health Information Provider," explores self-care for librarians whose work in "building the bridge" is often emotionally demanding.

It is through honing important interpersonal skills for professional health reference practice and personal self-care strategies that librarians derive the deep gratification inherent in our most important, often critical, work.

Acknowledgments

This work was born from being in the trenches, so to speak, through interacting with patients and consumers every day. I've been very fortunate because there have always been others in the trenches with me, people whose knowledge, skills, and experience have enriched my own life and helped shape who I am—both in the library and outside of it. I'd like to acknowledge a few of them:

Thank you to my "right hand" at work, Linda Stahl, for your integrity and professionalism, your good judgment and commitment to our work. You bring a depth and dimension to life to which I aspire.

To the administration of Mid-Columbia Medical Center, for your unwavering support of my outside teaching and consulting activities and for understanding that nourishing each individual employee's dream helps the entire organization to grow and flourish.

To the staff and volunteers of Planetree Health Resource Center, who succeed every day in serving the members of our diverse community. You are the "hum" in the apt expression, "keep things just humming along."

To the MLA Books Panel and Neal-Schuman Publishers, especially Charles Harmon, for your support and for believing I could carry this project off. To my editors, Elizabeth Lund, Paul Seeman, and Kathy Blake, who each had a hand in this book, for your expert guidance.

To my husband, Dan, my mentor and muse, my personal editor in chief. I'm grateful for your patience while I crafted this small book. In all things, you are my brilliant champion.

To the many patients, consumers, students, and colleagues I've had the pleasure to meet and interact with over the years, thank you for teaching me what it means to be a consumer health librarian.

Chapter 1

Professional Practice: Understanding and Reaching Out to the Health Information Seeker

"I have relapsing polychondritis. Are there any specialty clinics for this disorder?"

"I was teaching in Hong Kong and became ill. The doctor over there gave me these pills. Can you help me find out what they're for?"

"What can I do to reduce edema in addition to taking the diuretic pills my doctor has prescribed for me? Is there any special diet I can follow or herbs I can use?"

"I have stage III prostate cancer and my doctor has asked me to participate in a clinical trial. He's given me some information about it, but I'm wondering, how ill does the treatment really make you and how much time does it add to your life? I'm wondering if it's worth it . . ."

These are all real-life examples of the very pointed, sophisticated questions consumers are asking in libraries today. Such questions clearly indicate that many consumers are partners with their healthcare providers and taking ownership of their health concerns. How do we, as information professionals, support them in this meaningful endeavor?

Librarians are trained to be a bridge between an identified information need and the corresponding information resources that address that need. In providing consumer health information, we become a bridge in a broader sense: yes, a link between information need and resource, but also a tangible source of support for individuals in their process of research and discovery. Our supportive role stems from the fact that individuals seeking consumer health information are often in a personal dilemma. The need for sound information isn't just about understanding the disease and deciding among treatments; it also encompasses the *personal* impact of the illness: the individual's fear, uncertainty, and desire for resolution and hope. In addition to producing resources and materials that address the individual's query, information delivery requires understanding the psychology of healthcare consumers, which we will begin to explore in this chapter.

How Consumer Health Reference Requests Differ from Other Reference Requests

Most reference work is a very intellectual process. Many times we don't know how the information will be used; if we do know, it's typically for pleasure, personal growth, or to meet a business or school project deadline. In health reference, the stakes are higher. Often the results are discussed with healthcare providers or put to personal use. We see the human face of medical diagnoses, and in doing so we must confront our own fears about sickness, and ultimately, death. Coupling the emotional aspects of the patrons' illnesses with their desire for health information makes this work difficult. We are called into a deeper relationship with our patrons, and many times find ourselves perplexed or unprepared.

Consumer health reference questions take a variety of forms. You may be helping an individual who has recently been diagnosed or who is undergoing diagnostic tests. You may be assisting a family member who is coping with a loved one's illness. Sometimes you'll be working with a person who just wants to stay healthy. And of course you will confront the bane of all reference requests: the student who is writing a health paper. Each of these individuals brings special needs to the reference encounter, requiring compassionate reference work—a term not often used in librarianship.

Compassionate reference work starts with accepting the responsibility of being privileged with users' most intimate fears and information needs. It requires professional sensitivity, which we cultivate by using a holistic approach to the individual: Who is depending upon this person? Does the person have a family? Is he or she working, unemployed, or retired? Does he or she volunteer? Does the person live independently, or is he or she in need of shelter?

When we think of the patron as an individual, someone with family connections, who contributes to our world or is in need of assistance, we reflect upon an important truth: what we do matters.

Common Emotions among Consumer Health Information Seekers and Appropriate Responses

There are a number of common emotions among consumer health information seekers. Once we become familiar with them, we're able to employ strategies to address them. By doing so, we move past them to the heart of the person's visit: the actual reference request or information need.

Typically, individuals will want to tell you their "story"—how they found out about their illness or how they were diagnosed. This is especially true if they or someone they care about has recently been diagnosed with a serious disease, medical problem, or condition. Relating their story to you has an important purpose. Their storytelling is a form of processing their healthcare experience and all the different emotions and feelings that go along with it. Storytelling helps people make sense of their new reality by retelling it, sometimes over and over again.

It is vital for you as a professional to be at home with the many different feelings a user expresses. Characteristically, there may be expressions of vulnerability or helplessness or, at the other extreme, irritability or even outright anger. Remember, too, individuals seeking health information may simply not be feeling good; it may be hard for them to communicate or concentrate. They may express anxiety or worry.

In responding to these different emotions, keep one crucial thing in mind: these individuals are truly *not* themselves. People under stress act and cope differently, as do people who are grieving. They don't process information well. Often they are trying to gain some control over a world that suddenly seems completely out of control. Their visit to the library is extremely important. By researching their illness or condition, they are seeking to regain a measure of control, and thus reduce their burden through knowledge and understanding.

Your solution? Show you are in touch with and care about their feelings by making gentle eye contact and nodding appropriately as they speak. Listen attentively to their story and convey genuine interest. Finally, and this is key, acknowledge what they are going through by stating, "I understand you've had a difficult time," or "I hear your frustration." Acknowledgment is central to the interaction because it tells the user, "I have heard you and I understand." Such validation calms the individual and signals you are entering into a partnership with this person. For many individuals it will be an ongoing relationship as they make their way through the life adjustments and the treatments required by their new reality. After acknowledging their feelings, gently steer them to the purpose of their library visit by asking, "How can I help you while you are in the library?" Or "What do you need from the library today?"

> *Ellen was at the reference desk. A middle-aged woman approached her and smiled meekly. "How may I help you?" Ellen asked.*
>
> *"Oh, I don't know where to begin. I can't believe this. One minute my husband and I are planning our*

vacation and the next minute we are sitting in the doctor's office and he's saying my husband has lung cancer. He just had a little cough and we wanted to have it checked out before our trip." The woman starts to cry. "I know he smoked but he tried so hard to quit. The doctors are doing everything they can. They are talking about surgery and chemo. I don't know what they mean by stage IV. This can't be happening. He's too young. We're too young. We have so many decisions to make. I can't let my husband know how upset I am. He just can't handle it right now. He's trying to be brave but I just can't believe this."

Ellen comes out from behind the reference desk, offers the woman a tissue, and gently says, "I'm so sorry. I understand how difficult this must be." Several seconds pass while the woman weeps quietly and Ellen stands nearby. Then Ellen says softly, "There are so many things you need to think about. I'll be here to help you as you go through this. What is it you most want to find out about today? What information can I get for you or help you find while you are here?"

At this, the woman composes herself and says slowly, "I think I need a good overview of lung cancer to start with. Yes, I think that would be good. I mean, we don't really know anything about this." She seems relieved that she has begun the process of understanding this disease.

Common Concerns of Consumer Health Information Seekers and Appropriate Responses

In order to provide responsive service, we need to be proactive by anticipating common concerns or worries that individuals seeking health information often share. The most typical concerns—financial hardship, lack of self-confidence in conducting personal health research, Internet frustration, and, paradoxically, fear of physician reaction for researching personal health problems—are discussed here.

Financial and Insurance Concerns

Individuals with financial needs are everywhere. Healthcare today founders in a financial quagmire: declining or inadequate insurance coverage, high deductibles and co-pays, or a complete lack of insurance coverage. A Center on Budget and Policy Priorities report states that, according to 2005 U.S. Census Bureau data, 46.6 million Americans—or almost 16 percent of the population—lack healthcare insurance. Particularly noteworthy is that the percentage of Americans who are uninsured rose because the number of people with employer-provided health insurance benefits declined (Center on Budget and Policy Priorities, 2006). Lack of health insurance is compounded by other financial woes, such as climbing household debt in relation to disposable income (American Bankruptcy Institute, 2007). Of recent note, being able to afford prescription drugs is a huge challenge for many individuals. A Kaiser Family Foundation report, *Prescription Drug Trends*, points out the adverse effects of lack of prescription drug insurance coverage: "A 2005 survey found that uninsured adults are twice as likely as insured adults to say that they or a family member cut pills, did not fill a prescription, or skipped medical treatment in the past year because of the cost" (Kaiser Family Foundation, 2007). Workers, prevented from working while they are undergoing treatment, often feel financial stress. Who will pay the bills and put food on the table? Financial pressures are an additional burden for those suffering ill health.

Your solution? Normalize the individual's financial fears and provide a directory of available assistance. Don't wait to be asked; offer. Say something like, "We have this financial help guide I'd like to share with you because many people need support as they go through their illness."

In the financial guide, include information about local, state, and federal programs that assist people needing aid for healthcare goods and services. Include free clinics, clinics with sliding scale fees, affordable options for healthcare insurance, prescription drug assistance, help for obtaining assistive technology devices, and any other potentially useful information you can pull together. This can be a print guide or a Web site you develop. For inspiration, visit the Patient Advocate Foundation: www.patientadvocate. org and click on "PAF publications." Additional material may be found in the sample Financial Toolkit, Exhibit 5-1, included in Chapter 5.

Also, share information about ADA—the Americans with Disabilities Act—because many people don't realize illnesses, such as cancer, are protected in the workplace under the Act. Helpful information on ADA is covered in Exhibit 5-2, also in Chapter 5.

Concerns about Health and Medical Information

Anxiety about personal health and medical information retrieval skills plagues many users. Even in the twenty-first century, some people lack self-confidence in their ability to find information on their diagnosis or medical topic. According to the National Center for Education Statistics, 22 percent of U.S. adults have basic health literacy and another 14 percent have below basic health literacy, meaning they may range from being nonliterate in English to being able to understand *simple* information in documents or in working one-step problems (Kutner et al., 2006). Simply put, one-third of the U.S. population cannot understand most of the available health literature.

It's important to remember that both the history and language of medicine have their roots in secrecy. Medicine was handed down for generations among "medicine men" or apprentices who were chosen for their special healing abilities. No one else was privy to these secrets. Medical words are rooted in Latin, a language not very accessible for most people today. Despite "plain language" initiatives in healthcare to improve patient understanding, in the reality of day-to-day practice, medical jargon is still predominant. Physicians still talk in a "code" that few patients can understand.

When people visit the library, our approach is: teach as we go. Offer assistance but be aware that people may enter the consumer health library, especially if it is located within a hospital, with "white-coat expectations"—the belief that they will need to wait for service or for someone to initiate a transaction. Why? Because typically this is how they are treated within other areas of the healthcare system: medical procedures, exams, etc. *are performed on them.* As librarians, we want to inform people that *all* libraries are "hands-on." Then, we help them become proficient by teaching them how to use the different resources we have available.

> *A young mother enters the hospital's consumer health library with her baby in tow. She sees the staff is busy so she finds a seat and waits. After a while, Dana, a staff member, approaches her and says, "Are you waiting for someone or is there something I can help you with today?"*
>
> *The young woman says, "Oh, yes. Thank you. I just didn't know where to start. My pediatrician says my baby has [pulls a note out of her purse] 'seborrheic dermatitis' and I'm just so worried about her. I wanted to find out about it but I'm not even sure I know how to spell it."*
>
> *"If you like, I can show you how to search two Web sites that have great information on baby and child health issues," Dana replies. "These Web sites have what we call quality information—information you can trust—because they're run by reputable medical organizations. The information is written by medical experts and is very current. One of the sites has a medical dictionary— often a great place to start when looking something up for the first time. Shall I show you?"*

"Oh, I'd love that. Yes, thank you so much!"

Dana walks with the young mother to one of the computer stations and says, "I'm going to have you sit at the computer and I will talk you through how to use these Web sites. Are you okay with that?"

"You bet!" the woman replies, settling her baby in its baby carrier next to her on the floor as she sits down at the computer.

Concerns about Internet Reliability

The flip side of this is the net-savvy user who is frustrated with the Internet. There is an overwhelming amount of information available—some good, some not so good. According to a 2000 Pew Internet & American Life Project Report, "Eighty-six percent of health seekers . . . are concerned about getting information from an unreliable source online" (Fox and Rainie, 2000). Users typically don't understand the construct of the Internet or search order retrieval and how factors such as the placement of paid advertising affect a search. They just "Google it" and find themselves inundated with thousands of hits to sort through without knowing which sites offer trustworthy information. In fact, a 2006 Pew Internet & American Life Project Report stated, "Most respondents who searched for healthcare information online used search engines" (Fox, 2006). Furthermore, 75 percent of online health information seekers "say they check the source and date 'only sometimes,' 'hardly ever,' or 'never,' which translates to about 85 million Americans gathering health advice online without consistently examining the quality indicators of the information they find" (Fox, 2006).

Your solution? Teach the basics of sound Internet searching. Include the importance of reliability, credibility, and currency of health information. Explain bias. Explain the meaning of Web site extensions: .edu/.gov/.net/.com. Set up user-friendly search stations with subject links to trusted sites. Remember that when you bookmark Web sites or refer people to them, less is more. It's easy to overwhelm someone who is feeling vulnerable, so keep the number of Web sites you suggest to two or three. If these sites meet the criteria of quality health Web sites, they will link to other helpful Web sites.

> *Melissa is at the reference desk when the telephone rings. An agitated caller says, "I've been searching the Internet and it's driving me crazy. I want to find out some information on Naproxen and I just keep getting these Web sites trying to sell me drugs. I have arthritis and my doctor is suggesting I try this for my pain and I want to read about it, but this is ridiculous. Can you help me?"*
>
> *"I know how frustrated you must be. Searching the Web can be very time consuming. Yes, I can help you. I'm going to guide you to a Web site that has credible information on both Naproxen and arthritis and contains no advertising. Does that sound good? Okay, please point your browser to . . ."*

Concerns about Physician Reaction or Reprimand

Even though patient-centered care is gaining ground in health-care facilities across the United States, another common concern of health information seekers arises simply from fear. Patrons may fear their diagnosis, certainly, but they also may fear physician reaction or reprimand for researching their health concern. They may worry that such research could be viewed as "second-guessing" the physician's authority. Others are concerned that discussing their research will take up too much of their physician's time with questions, again upsetting the delicate doctor-patient relationship.

In the book *Patients as Partners: How to Involve Patients and Families in Their Own Care* (Joint Commission, 2006), it's noted that, on average, physicians listen to their patients for 18 to 23 seconds before interrupting. Of course, the interruption disrupts two-way communication vital to a healthy doctor-patient relationship. Patients treated abruptly are not apt to question a physician or even engage in much of a dialogue. Because patient safety suffers as a result, the Joint Commission's National Patient Safety Goals puts "clear communication" on the front burner of the nation's health quality criteria as a means to improve both patient safety and quality of care (Joint Commission, 2008). While there is a concerted effort underway to improve doctor-patient communication, and many consumer-oriented books and materials have been published on this topic, real change takes time. In the meantime, it's important to be aware of this common concern of health information seekers and helpful ways you can address it in the library setting.

Your solution? Stock your consumer health library with consumer or patient advocacy materials (see Exhibit 1-1, Patient Advocacy Materials), such as "Talking with Your Doctor . . ." or various versions of a "Patient's Bill of Rights." As suggested earlier, always encourage your library users to share the health information they find with their healthcare provider.

Exhibit 1-1. Patient Advocacy Materials

American Hospital Association Management Advisory: A Patient's Bill of Rights. 1992. Chicago, IL: American Hospital Association. www.patienttalk.info/AHA-Patient_Bill_of_Rights.htm.

Quick Tips—When Talking with Your Doctor. AHRQ Publication No. 01-0040a, May 2002. Agency for Healthcare Research and Quality, Rockville, MD. www.ahrq.gov/consumer/quicktips/doctalk.pdf.

Talking with Your Doctor: A Guide for Older People. NIH Publication No. 05-3452 August, 2005. National Institute on Aging. www.niapublications.org/pubs/talking/Talking_with_Your_Doctor.pdf.

> On duty at the reference desk, Katie is approached by an older gentleman. He looks a little shy, so Katie greets him warmly and says, "How may I help you today?"
>
> "Well, gee, I'm not sure," the man says, shaking his head back and forth. "My doctor says I have early-stage prostate cancer and he wants me to have surgery. But I don't know . . . I'm only 68 years old. I just wonder, are there any other options? I know I shouldn't be here and try to be my own doctor. In fact, my own doctor doesn't know I'm here—it might upset him if he knew. But, you know, this is my life and my wife and I were talking and just wondering, is there anything else they can do? It just scares me—the idea of surgery and geez, the list of problems you can have. A mile long! I don't know, I guess if I read more about it I might be okay, but I just wonder, are there any other options?"
>
> Katie walks around from behind the reference desk and says, "What you're doing is right. You're taking ownership of your care. Cancer is a very difficult diagnosis and there are many decisions to make. It's important to be as well informed as possible. There is a lot of current information about early-stage prostate cancer, and actually, there are treatment options you will want to talk with your doctor about. Let's start with some prostate cancer–specific information, and then, if you like, we can look for some patient self-advocacy materials. Is that okay with you?"
>
> "Oh, yes, by all means! Thank you so much," the man says.

Understanding common concerns of people seeking health information prepares you to think about and develop appropriate ways of responding. Where fear, confusion, worry, anxiety, frustration, sadness, and disbelief are evident, it's your compassion, coupled with professional confidence, that provides a safe and reassuring environment. Meeting the individual's basic need for affirmation of his or her feelings allows you to steer the conversation to the reference encounter—the patient's real purpose in visiting the library.

Promoting and Marketing Your Library's Services

In our information-drenched society there are still some rare diagnoses and conditions for which it is difficult to find credible information. Reference librarians are acutely aware that health reference requests are often for very specific information.

Your solution? Reassure patrons that you, the librarian, have the expertise to find elusive health information. In marketing your library's services, publicize the depth and scope of your collection and *never miss an opportunity* to sell your most important asset: your staff's professional expertise. Publicize your staff's ability to locate trustworthy information. Clearly convey staff expertise in your marketing efforts. Market their highly developed search retrieval skills, which enable them to filter through the mass of electronic information and zero in on specific, accurate details—a critical skill where health information is concerned. In developing ads or brochures, use a hook or tagline that people can identify with so they think of you in their time of need. Here are a few ideas, although your public relations department will want to tailor such an ad campaign to your community:

- Is finding information on your diagnosis like looking for a needle in a haystack? Call XXX Health Library. Our staff knows how to zero in.

- When the world of medicine seems fuzzy, your medical librarian can help you see clearly! Call XXX-XXXX for help.

- Lost in the medical information maze? Let XXX health library amaze you with their sure sense of direction.

Think of this analogy: When people want their hair done, they go to a hair stylist. Similarly, when people want health information, they should call or visit a health information specialist.

There are a number of ways to market and promote your staff. One of the best is to participate in social and business club events by offering to give a presentation. Put together a creative program using PowerPoint that shows your library and discusses the services you provide. Plan time for a question-and-answer session. You can take this same program and customize it for patient support groups. Be sure to give concrete examples of how you can be helpful. Similarly, when promoting your library in any format, such as print or radio ads, tout your staff's expertise. Make sure your library bookmarks, flyers, or brochures mention that you have a staff of health information *specialists*. Ask permission to adequately stock and display these promotional items in key community locations, such as physician waiting rooms, health agency offices, hospital waiting areas, coffeehouse bulletin boards, and the like. Whenever you speak publicly, make sure you leave your audience with something to remember you by: a bookmark, a pen with the library logo, or a refrigerator magnet, for example.

You must also lay the groundwork with your area's healthcare providers to enlist their support and to promote yourself as a helpful and valuable resource to their medical practice. Contact clinic office managers and ask to give a brief (ten-minute) presentation about your services to their staff at one of their regular staff meetings. Typically, these meetings are early morning or over a lunch hour, so offer to bring food: muffins and juice for a morning meeting, pizza or deli sandwiches for lunch. This is a crucial step to getting in the door. Perhaps there should be a medical office adage, "If you feed them, they will come." Show the staff how you can be an asset to them—a help to their patients and their practice in general. Explain your role as a librarian in providing health information and reassure them that librarians do not dispense advice or aid in patients' decision making. Librarians simply provide information from trusted sources in response to a specific request. Make it clear that you encourage library users to discuss information they obtain in the library with their physician. Share studies with the doctors showing that both informed patients and those who have good communication with their doctor are less likely to sue for malpractice (Levinson, 1994) and more likely to follow their doctor's recommendations (Spiegel and Kavaler, 1997). You may want to offer a prescription-type pad (see Exhibit 1-2, Health Information Request) for clinic physicians or their assistants to fill out and give to their patients directing them to your library for more information. If you are part of a wired hospital or health system, you might request to have this form on the electronic medical record, prompting the physician to ask about health information needs and then automatically directing the request to the librarian for fulfillment.

Summary

In today's information-rich society and complex healthcare environment, being a consumer health librarian affords us the opportunity to serve people to the best of our professional capacity. It's true that we have the skills and tools to help health information consumers find the answers they seek but, just as importantly, we have an intrinsic need to *serve* others in a very meaningful way by anticipating their needs and providing practical responses. The tools and tips offered in this chapter help us to deepen our professional practice in a manner that is both responsible and responsive to each individual's unique health information concerns.

Of course, all this is for naught if people who need help finding health information are unaware of your expertise and desire to help. Promotion and outreach, to both your primary clientele as well as local healthcare providers, informs everyone of your ability to provide a trusted place to turn to during a personal time of uncertainty or a life-changing experience.

Exhibit 1-2. Health Information Request

Note: this is a two-sided form.

Library Name
Health Information Request
Library Street Address
City, Zip Code, Telephone Number/E-mail Address

Dear Health Library Staff:

Please help my patient find information on the following diagnosis:

_____

Include information on:

Overview——Treatment(s)——Diet ——
Exercise——Coping/Stress ——

Specific Medication(s) _____

Complications (specify) _____

Other_____

(see other side for pertinent information)

(side 2)

Patient's Name & Address _____

_____

Patient's Age___ Sex ___

Smoker___ Nonsmoker ___

Notes:

_____
Requesting Physician/Nurse Name

References

American Bankruptcy Institute. 2007. "News Room: Consumer Debt Is Consistent with Bankruptcy Filings." Alexandria, VA: ABI. (October 1). Available: www.abiworld.org/Content/NavigationMenu/NewsRoom/BankruptcyStatistics/Bankruptcy_Filings_1.htm.

Center on Budget and Policy Priorities. 2006. "The Number of Uninsured Americans Is at an All-Time High." Washington, DC: Center on Budget and Policy Priorities. (August 29). Available: www.cbpp.org/8-29-06health.htm.

Fox, Susannah. 2006. "Online Health Search 2006." Washington DC: Pew Internet & American Life Project. (October). Available: www.pewinternet.org.

Fox, Susannah, and Lee Rainie. 2000. "The Online Healthcare Revolution: How the Web Helps Americans Take Better Care of Themselves." Washington, DC: Pew Internet & American Life Project. (November). Available: www.pewinternet.org.

Joint Commission. 2006. *Patients as Partners: How to Involve Patients and Families in Their Own Care.* Oakbrook Terrace, IL: Joint Commission Resources.

Joint Commission. 2008. "National Patient Safety Goals." Available: http://www.jcipatientsafety.org/15148.

Kaiser Family Foundation. 2007. "Prescription Drug Trends." Menlo Park, CA: Kaiser Family Foundation. (May). Available: www.kff.org/rxdrugs/upload/3057_06.pdf.

Kutner, M., E. Greenberg, Y. Jin, and C. Paulsen. 2006. "The Health Literacy of America's Adults: Results from the 2003 National Assessment of Adult Literacy." National Center for Education Statistics, U.S. Department of Education. NCES 2006-483. (September).

Levinson, W. 1994. "Physician-Patient Communication: A Key to Malpractice Prevention." JAMA 272, no. 20 (November): 1619–1620.

Spiegel A. D., and F. Kavaler. 1997. "Better Patient Communications Mean Lower Liability Exposure." *Managed Care* 6, no. 8 (August): 119–124.

Chapter 2

Professional Interactions: Communication Guidelines and Strategies

Communication is tricky. Many of us remember playing the telephone game when we were growing up—whispering a message around a circle of friends and then laughing out loud when the final person relayed the message and, in comparing it to the first person's communication, everyone realized it was grossly distorted. In the reference setting, we want to minimize communication distortions. We must, in order to do our job. This chapter focuses on the importance of both nonverbal and verbal communication in the consumer health reference interaction.

Nonverbal Communication

A common perception is that verbal communication is all-important. Let's face it; we live in a culture that is constantly talking. Yet on a deeper level, we know that communication is more than mere words, hence the familiar saying, "Actions speak louder than words." An early researcher of body language, anthropologist Ray Birdwhistell, found that over 65 *percent* of communication is made nonverbally or without words (Pease and Pease, 2004). Researchers today continue to agree that the majority of communication is accomplished nonverbally. It is our posture, facial expression, tone of voice (or sounds that we make), and gestures that speak volumes to library users, yet many of us give this little thought. We put more emphasis on words, but words are only a small part of the communication picture.

We've discussed the different vulnerabilities people bring to the health reference encounter in Chapter 1. In order to put people at ease, competent communication is essential. One key to communicating with anyone is congruency—our body language and our words must complement each other; they must be in sync. Your verbal and nonverbal clues will work together to project whether you are open-minded and approachable. For example, if someone walks up to the reference desk, and you say, "How can I help you?" without making eye contact, it's doubtful that the patron will believe you are truly interested in assisting, and he or she may just walk away.

Basic Nonverbal Communication Strategies

The good news is that there are some basic nonverbal communication strategies you can employ for successful patron interaction. The first, as mentioned above, is to make good eye contact. In order to connect with other people, you must look them in the eye. We're not talking about staring, but comfortable eye contact. Unless this is a cultural taboo, you have more credibility with others when you make eye contact (Pease and Pease, 2004).

Second, develop awareness of your facial expression and adjust it, if necessary. For example, if the patron you're helping reflected your face back to you, just as if you were looking in a mirror, what would you see? Would it be someone open and inviting, a calm, friendly face? Or are your lips pursed and is your brow furrowed? Then ask yourself, "Which librarian would I want to approach?" We all know looks can kill, and in the library, they can kill the desire to request professional assistance on a difficult topic such as a person's health.

Third, what are your stance and body language telling your patron? Do you present yourself as a fortress or a summer cottage? Maybe you think it's comfortable to cross your arms over your chest, yet this pose signifies a very self-protective and defensive attitude. If your arms are relaxed, down at your sides, your palms open, this signifies sincerity and receptivity (Pease and Pease, 2004). Of the two examples, the first one repels a user; the second offers an invitation.

Finally, *hear* tones of voice. By listening intently to the patron, you will be able to hear anger, frustration, fear, sorrow, and sometimes, blessedly, joy. Tuning in to the patron's tone of voice gives you a reference point to orient your response. You want to respond professionally, of course, but you must acknowledge the patron's emotions and reply accordingly.

The flip side of hearing tones of voice is to hear *your own*. A calm voice is most soothing to someone in crisis. Do not let the private irritations of your day—the argument you had with your spouse, child, or significant other, or the frustration you feel because you had a flat tire on the way to work—influence your tone of voice while assisting your patrons. These sounds carry meaning: If your tone of voice sounds angry, uninterested, impatient, or patronizing, you won't connect with your patrons; furthermore, you've given them good reason not to trust you during their time of crisis. Imagine a time you dealt with bad customer service. More than likely you still remember the tone of voice the person used and how off-putting it was.

Vocal sounds may also intimidate library users. Most in our profession are familiar with the unflattering stereotype of the librarian "shushing" clients and the poor public image we have suffered because of it. Clicking and tsking noises, harrumphing, and audible nostril breathing send a strong nonverbal message of annoyance. Because people look for synergy between words, actions, and nonverbal communication, it won't matter that you have told your library user, "I can help you"; such sounds indicate agitation or superiority. If you sigh your way through the reference transaction, not only will it be an unpleasant experience for the library user, but also he or she will not put much credibility in you as a resource. Voice tone and sounds matter, so work hard to keep yours even and respectful.

Utilizing Self-awareness to Strengthen Communication Skills

We must use our self-awareness to be conscious of the nonverbal messages we send library patrons, then apply this awareness to make adjustments. Learning any new skill or technique takes practice and this includes changing the way we present ourselves to others. As you go about your day, ask yourself, "What am I saying to others through my gestures, my tone of voice, my body stance?" When you realize you are drumming your fingers (impatient), slouching (bored), or standing stiff as a board (scared or aloof), for example, use this knowledge to soften your body language. By softening any cold, hard features, our warm body language makes it more likely a vulnerable health information seeker will approach us for help.

As people visit the library, practice the art of acknowledgment. If you're sitting at your desk, set things aside, look up, and greet them. Shift forward in your seat a bit, to indicate both your interest in helping them and your desire to hear their request.

Exhibit 2-1. Nonverbal Communication Resources

Books

Mehrabian, Albert. 2007. *Nonverbal Communication.* Piscataway, NJ: Transaction.

Pease, Allan, and Barbara Pease. 2004. *The Definitive Book of Body Language.* New York: Bantam.

Web Sites

Exploring Nonverbal Communication. University of California at Santa Cruz. http://nonverbal.ucsc.edu.

The Nonverbal Dictionary of Gestures, Signs & Body Language Cues. By David Givens, PhD. Spokane, Washington: Center for Nonverbal Studies Press. Available: http://members.aol.com/nonverbal2/diction1.htm.

Finally, check the reference environment for clues signaling that it's all right to have a private conversation. Make sure the reference desk is free of clutter and the reference desk chair faces the public. Is the desk itself a hindrance? If so, challenge your staff to come up with creative solutions to minimize its impact on the exchange of confidential information. If you are in a very busy arena, consider walking the patron to a private area to conduct a more in-depth reference interview. Come around from behind the desk and offer assistance. By taking just a few steps away from the reference desk, you've created an air of privacy.

Much has been studied and written about nonverbal communication. See Exhibit 2-1, Nonverbal Communication Resources, to learn more.

Verbal Communication

We know people experiencing a health crisis are stressed, and people under stress are truly not themselves. People in crisis feel they have lost control of their world, and in fact, this is true. Their desire is to restore order and balance and one way to do so is to learn about their problem or condition. Your demeanor as the reference librarian will either help your library users or make things worse. We have discussed the importance of congruity between verbal and nonverbal communication. When it comes to words, this is where the art of compassionate neutrality comes into play.

Compassionate Neutrality

Compassionate neutrality is the art of absorbing the full context of what a patron tells you without judgment, criticism, or pity. Compassionate neutrality means hearing what the user tells you, acknowledging his or her feelings, and then doing your job. It is a professional expression of the human dimension in the reference interview.

In speaking with library patrons who have health questions, your personal comfort zone may be tested. Knowing what pushes your buttons or what really gets under your skin, as well as where you are most vulnerable, is essential in order to maintain neutrality. This is especially true because most people seeking health information begin by telling you their medical story. As people tell you their medical story—what their diagnosis is, how long it took to get their test results, how difficult their life has been, how unfair this condition is, how difficult it will be to pay for their treatment or care, whether a complementary therapy is a magic bullet, and so on—you will be privy to information that may anger you, make you incredibly sad, or perhaps leave you feeling as if a great injustice has occurred. As we learned in Chapter 1, this storytelling gives meaning to the patrons' experiences and is very important for processing their new reality. Their need to be heard and understood is real.

By practicing compassionate neutrality through keeping your feelings in check, you become a safe harbor in the library users' health storm. Just as their world is being tossed by unexpected waves, they will look to you as an anchor, something solid to depend upon and will come to you for help in finding answers to their health dilemmas.

As you listen to someone's medical story, acknowledge what the individual is feeling without adding meaning to it by expressing your own emotions. For example, if someone is upset and venting frustration at the healthcare system for its slowness, listen quietly for a while, then gently break in, and say, "I hear you are upset about how long it took for your test results to come back. I'm sure it was very hard to wait." Then steer the conversation back to the reason for the visit, adding, "Now, how can I help you here in the library today?" or "Now, what brings you to the library today?"

> *An elderly gentleman enters the library and appears greatly upset. When Esme, the reference librarian, approaches him, she smiles and says, "May I help you?" He replies, rather loudly and distraught, "Help me? God, yes! I can't get any answers from my doctor. He's done all these tests and I still don't know a thing! Why won't he talk to me? These doctors*

today just don't take the time to tell you anything! But, oh, they'll take your money!"

Moving closer, Esme says, "I understand you are upset and frustrated with your doctor and the whole process of waiting for a diagnosis. It's agonizing and I understand. I'm so sorry you are in that uncomfortable place, but what brings you to the library today? What can we do while you are here to help you feel better? Is there anything in particular you want to learn about?"

With that, the gentleman grumbles a bit and then says, "Well, he told me I needed an MRI. I have no idea what this is. I just want to know what this is, what it does to you, how it works."

Esme says, "I can definitely help you with that. We have several options—would you like to see a movie, read about it, see a picture, or all of the above?"

"Well, if it isn't too much trouble, all of the above!" replies the gentleman, who now appears much more relaxed.

Avoid Medical Jargon

Another verbal communication key is to keep your sentences short and clear—no medical jargon, no impressive repertoire of technical medical information. Use words that are highly accessible and that people understand, language referred to in the literature on health literacy as "living room language." Many studies have confirmed that anxious, fearful people, such as someone under the stress of a challenging diagnosis or family crisis, have difficulty processing information (Millar, 2005). This can be especially true for patrons who have a different cultural background or whose native language is not English. A consumer health reference interview across cultural perspectives with someone who has limited English-speaking ability can be quite challenging. Similarly, individuals with impaired hearing also require special consider-

Exhibit 2-2. Communication Tips for Special Reference Interviews

Patrons with Limited English-Speaking Ability

❑ **Speak slowly,** using short, simple sentences. Enunciate clearly, using proper English. Avoid using jargon or acronyms.

❑ **Face the individual** and speak directly to him or her.

❑ **Use pictures** or illustrations.

❑ **Be patient** and repeat if necessary.

❑ **Have a language identification list** or flash cards available so individuals can identify their native language. For example, offer a list or a flash card with "I speak Chinese" written on it in Chinese and translated into English.

❑ **Call Interpreter Services** for support, if you have such a service available.

❑ **Use the universal "okay?"** to ascertain understanding. Don't be afraid to tell the individual, "I'm sorry. I do not understand." Try again.

Patrons with Impaired Hearing

❑ **Speak slowly.** Enunciate clearly. Face the individual so he or she can see your lips.

❑ **Shorten the distance** between the two of you. Stand still as you speak.

❑ **Speak loudly,** but don't shout.

❑ **Choose different words** if the individual doesn't understand you. Some words are easier for the individual to recognize.

❑ **Move the individual** away from areas where there is a lot of background noise—such as a busy information desk—so he or she can concentrate on your conversation.

ation. Medical jargon has no place in these types of interviews. Refer to Exhibit 2-2, Communication Tips for Special Reference Interviews, for helpful suggestions.

It's clear that employing good verbal and nonverbal communication strategies will help ensure that library patrons won't be playing the telephone game when they interact with us. The skills and practices discussed in this section will help minimize communication distortion and will serve you well as you conduct the reference interview.

Reference Interview Techniques

For many librarians, this section will be a brief review. There may be new material here, but the intention is to cover the basics of sound reference interview techniques. In library school, we learned that open questions elicit information. Used wisely, they work well to draw an individual out and determine the real information sought. The basics still work: who, what, when, where, why, and how. Closed questions narrow the focus of the interview and wrap things up. Closed questions elicit yes-or-no answers. Closed questions confirm that you understand the information need or have met the user's needs. The following are examples of open questions:

- **Who** is the information for?

- **What** is the exact diagnosis? Note: When patrons don't know, STOP. Encourage them to contact their doctor's office and come back when they have the diagnosis. Suggest that they talk with the nurse, because most people don't want to "bother" their doctor, and note that HIPAA privacy rules apply; they may have to identify themselves in some unique way. *Many* medical words sound alike but have drastically different implications for an individual. The last thing you want is someone going home with the wrong medical information. Don't guess or surmise; if in doubt, don't proceed.

Example: ascariasis sounds very similar to acariasis. One is a disease caused by the parasitic worm *Ascaris lumbricoides*; the other is a disease, usually a skin infection, caused by mites.

- **Where** have you looked already?

- **When** are you having the test done?

- **How** much information do you want?

- **Why** do you need this information? For a school report or personal use?

Here are some examples of closed questions:

- **Is** this what you are looking for?

- **Has** the procedure already been done?

- **Can** you spell the diagnosis for me?

- **Does** this meet your needs?

- **Will** you need treatment information?

Define Unfamiliar Terms

Remember to define unfamiliar terms such as acronyms, which are often used in medicine. For example, does AMA refer to Against Medical Advice or the American Medical Association? Make sure you have the correct spelling of a diagnosis—systemic lupus erythamatosis or systemic lupus erythematosus? (it's the latter one)—so you'll be able to search and retrieve accurate information. Also, if a diagnosis is new to you, check the definition to give you a solid foundation for your research efforts. For example, you may think you know the definition of cryobiology. Perhaps you believe it is the science of crying, when in fact, after looking it up, you discover it is the science of dealing with the effect of low temperatures on biological systems!

Utilize the Talk-Back Technique

Be honest, yet reassuring, to your patron if a topic or diagnosis is new to you. Use the parrot, or talk-back technique, to summarize the information request: "I understand you are interested in finding out how radiation therapy is used to treat early-stage endometrial cancer. Is that correct?" And finally, share your research strategy with your patron—teach as you go, to empower your users for their future health information needs. For example, as you begin your search, explain, "So you're looking for information on normal glucose levels for a blood test you are having done tomorrow? Let's look at a Web site called Labtestsonline.org."

Handling Unpleasant News

In the course of our work, we may discover that the illness or medical condition a patron is inquiring about has a poor prognosis. We may not know whether the patron is aware of the expected outcome and this realization may catch us off guard. It's important to remember to practice compassionate neutrality in this situation—to maintain our composure and professionalism.

So how do we respond? First, ask whether the physician has explained the diagnosis. You may be surprised when the answer is "yes." If this is the case, then proceed with the reference interview and gently help locate the information. You may want to offer the individual a comfortable place to sit while you bring appropriate materials. Regardless of the information you share, always encourage your patrons to discuss it with their healthcare providers. Explain that the information found in the library may or may not apply to their unique clinical case and only their doctors can make this judgment. Let the individuals know you are available if they require further assistance and check back after a while to see how they're doing.

It is most agonizing when the individual has not yet learned of or does not comprehend a poor prognosis. You have important knowledge that the individual lacks, and this can be uncomfortable. You may know that the typical course of the disease is to become progressively worse, severely change a person's quality of life, or even be ultimately fatal. In this very difficult situation, you will want to first soften the impact of the information you are about to share. You are using the "cushion approach," preparing the individual to hear bad news. This is never easy, so I suggest you develop a script—words you are comfortable with that will come naturally for you when you must use them. Remember that you, too, may be stressed in this situation. The last thing you want is to be struggling for the right words, so choose words for your script that you can easily recall—something sincere yet memorable. Practice your script when you are *not* in a stressful situation, so you will be comfortable and familiar with it and will be able to employ it when you need it most.

You might say something like this: "I'm concerned about the nature of the information you'll find about this condition, because it may be distressing or hard to grasp. I'm sure you'll want to discuss this with your doctor. You're welcome to take the information with you, so you can do so." Explain that the information you are sharing is "a textbook case" and that "as a unique individual, the information may or may not apply" to the person. Emphasize to patrons that their physician understands their complete medical history and symptoms and thus will be able to explain whether or not the information is truly relevant to them.

As you share the information about their diagnosis, also offer supportive measures. This applies equally to those who've answered "yes" and those who've answered "no" to the question, "Has your doctor explained the diagnosis?" Be prepared to listen and offer a private area for the individual to be alone for a brief period of time, if possible. Small comfort measures are often welcomed—a cup of hot tea, a cool drink of water, a box of tissues. These small kindnesses are appreciated in such a stressful situation. Share local support group information if appropriate; many patients find consolation and solidarity in their participation. If your library is within a hospital, you may have social workers or pastoral care team members whom you can call for just these types of interactions. They are highly trained to respond to patrons who are shocked when the gravity of their diagnosis is revealed. One caveat: please seek permission first from your library patron before calling for help. They've had enough surprises for one day. You might suggest, "I know you've just received some very difficult news. We have a chaplain on staff whom I can call for you. Would you like me to do that?" Whatever you say or do, let your compassion and empathy come through. It's important to recognize that compassion is not pity, but nonjudgmental understanding.

E-mail and Virtual Reference Guidelines

Much has been written in the library literature about e-mail and virtual reference service. A few caveats should be remembered when providing consumer health information through these electronic formats. A clear policy is essential and is the foundation for any service provision. Make sure your policy states what you will (and conversely won't) provide via electronic reference, the hours the service is available, the expected response time, other options for users to obtain reference help, and privacy cautions.

Users believe they are anonymous when sending electronic reference requests and, therefore, they may be emboldened. They may even cross the line of appropriateness. Individuals will share lengthy personal health histories and the range of different specialists they have tried or are currently seeing. They may rant about the care they've experienced, or share their despair with you and let you know you are their last, best hope.

Communication differs in e-reference because you cannot use nonverbal clues to assist you in the reference interview. There is no easy way to discern a user's emotional state or respond to it, unless the user shares that information in writing. Just as in the face-to-face encounter, you must set boundaries about what type of assistance a librarian can provide. When e-mail users ask you to interpret information, to make sense of their medical history by offering a diagnosis, or to suggest the right "next step" for them to take, you must be clear that you cannot do so, for that is outside the scope of your practice as a librarian.

Educate E-users

It's also important to educate users that e-mail messages are not private and, in fact, are discoverable evidence in lawsuits. You do need users to be clear about what information they are seeking, but you don't want them to pour out every intimate detail of their medical condition or diagnosis to you. Post guidelines on how to use your e-mail service. For example, "In order to serve you best, please answer the following questions regarding your request for health information:

- Who is the information for, yourself or a loved one?

- What is the patient's age and gender?

- What is the diagnosis or medical condition?

- What type of information is desired?: diagnosis, treatment, specialized treatment centers, coping/lifestyle, stress reduction, caregiver support, nutrition, complementary (or alternative) therapies, other (specify)"

You might list the questions on an electronic form that users can fill out and submit. You'll also want to post your timeline for responding to e-mail inquiries. Because people often ask for health information in response to a crisis, please be sensitive to the immediacy of the request and set reasonable response times.

Virtual Reference

Although virtual reference is real-time service, the same guidelines apply. Be clear about the discoverable nature of electronic communication. Ask the user need-to-know questions rather than soliciting extraneous information in your online conversation. Be kind yet firm regarding your inability to interpret how the information you retrieve applies to the medical situation being queried. Always suggest that users discuss the health information you've identified with their healthcare provider.

Some users will persist in e-mailing you about the same health issue when you have exhausted all your research capabilities. In this case, be clear that you have nothing else to offer. You might say, "I'm sorry, but I can no longer offer you assistance because I have exhausted my limited expertise on researching this topic." If you can, offer another avenue for the user to pursue. "Perhaps the reference staff at Cascade University Medical Center has additional resources." Make your closing statement firm: "Thank you for using Mill Creek Hospital's Virtual Reference Service."

As discussed earlier, the policies and procedures defining the scope of your e-reference service should be developed and posted up front. Here's what can happen if you fail to do so. How would you respond to the following?

> *"My name is Clara. I am 51, with a diagnosis of bipolar II, rapid cycling, and borderline personality disorder. I have made multiple suicide attempts. Mental illness runs in my family. Both my mom and my niece have bipolar and also have attempted suicide. With my family history, would my diagnosis also be bipolar IV—bipolar with family history of bipolar?*
>
> *"I've been prescribed Ambien 60 mg (six 10 mg pills a day) and 20 mg Ativan as needed for anxiety and Klonopin 2 mg (3 x day). I've taken Ativan and Ambien for years. What long-term damages might I expect from being on such high dosages of Ativan and Ambien for so long? I did not realize that my medications were so dangerous but my short-term memory appears to be going and I've lost my ability to focus or concentrate.*
>
> *"I also have a question about my first violent suicide attempt last March, when I stabbed myself in the chest with a six-inch blade and took too many of my meds. I was rushed to the ER and survived. My doctor had previously put me on Nardil and had*

*recently increased the dose. Could the Nardil have
made my bipolar worse?"*

*"I would appreciate your professional opinion on
my bipolar, the long-term damages of Ambien and
Ativan, and whether you think Nardil triggered my
violent suicide attempt. Thank you."*

Suggested response:

*"I'm going to list some Web sites that may be of help
to you in finding answers to your questions. I am
a medical librarian, and, as such, cannot interpret
or make recommendations regarding your care.
However, I have located some Web sites that I think
will be useful to you."*

*"This first site is the HealthTalk on Bipolar
Disorders at www2.healthtalk.com/go/mental-health
/bipolar-disorder. From the Disease Basics box in the
center of the page, you can access the 'Our Experts
Answer Your Questions' feature . . ."*

Telephone Reference Guidelines

Where health information is concerned, telephone reference also
requires clear guidelines. Of course, you'll give factual information
over the telephone: a hospital's address, a support group meeting
time and location, whether or not you have a particular resource
in your collection. You'll want to encourage callers to visit the
library and its Web site. For homebound callers, you might suggest that they visit the library when they are able and direct them
to your library's Web site.

You may read a brief definition verbatim over the telephone, *if
you first ask the caller if the doctor has explained the diagnosis to them.*
You do not want to be put in the position of reading a definition
of a terminal illness over the telephone. As discussed in the section on handling unpleasant news, if the caller is uninformed, you
might say something like, "I'm so sorry, but I don't have time to

read this to you right now. I'm staffing the desk by myself and we are very busy. If you'll please give me your address, I'll send this definition to you in the mail. You may want to discuss it with your doctor and then you will have a copy to share with him or her." If the caller persists, then you'll want to employ the "cushion" approach discussed earlier (see the "Handling Unpleasant News" section). Reading the definition word-for-word, you'll want to make sure you have enough time to provide comfort to the caller. If at all possible, move to a private area so other library users are not disturbed by your end of the conversation.

Always give the caller the complete source of information and note that you are going to read exactly from the text. When you are finished reading, the caller may ask, "What does that mean?" Clarify that by law you cannot interpret the information. You might gently say, "I'm so sorry. I know you are trying to understand this information, but by law I cannot explain it or interpret it for you. Your doctor will know how to answer your questions, so you will want to contact him or her about this." Offer to mail the information so the caller can read it and share it with his or her healthcare provider.

Summary

For consumer health librarians, good communication—both verbal and nonverbal—is critical. It trumps all other skills necessary to perform our work, for without it, we have no way to interact with or relate to our patrons.

Whether interacting face-to-face in the library or via e-reference or telephone, solid communication is the key. Good communication requires that we present ourselves as approachable and competent. Good body language and clarity in spoken words are building blocks, but sensitivity to the user is paramount. We must have the skills and ability to use compassionate neutrality to gently discern the user's information needs and respond accordingly. And, perhaps most important, as consumer health librarians, we must have a desire to serve.

Additional Reading

Curry, Evelyn L. 2005. "The Reference Interview Revisited: Librarian-Patron Interaction in the Virtual Environment." *SIMILE: Studies in Media & Information Literacy Education 5, no. 1 (February)*. Available: *http://utpjournals.metapress*.com/ content/g03265637016/?p=7a01628ef784443989da98ae9c26 9b66&pi=10.

Eckwright, Gail, Tam Hoskisson, and Mike Pollastro. 1998. "Reference Etiquette: A Guide to Excruciatingly Correct Behavior." *American Libraries* (May): 42–45.

Sielski, Lester M. 1979. "Understanding Body Language." *Personnel and Guidance Journal* 57, no. 5: 238–242.

Straw, J. E. 2000. "A Virtual Understanding: Reference Interview and Question Negotiation in the Digital Age." *Reference and User Services Quarterly* 39, no. 4: 376–379.

References

Millar, Murray. 2005. "The Effects of Perceived Stress on Reactions to Messages Designed to Increase Health Behaviors." *Journal of Behavioral Medicine* 28, no. 5: 425–432.

Pease, Allan, and Barbara Pease. 2004. *The Definitive Book of Body Language*. New York: Bantam.

Chapter 3

Professional Ethics of Providing Health Information

Being a consumer health librarian has its special challenges. For example, what if you know the patron personally? This is especially difficult if you live in a small town or you are the only health librarian on staff. Fortunately, librarians operate under a code of ethics such as the Medical Library Association's Code of Ethics for Health Sciences Librarianship (Medical Library Association, 1994) and the American Library Association's Code of Ethics (American Library Association, 1995), both included at the end of this chapter (Appendix 3-1 and Appendix 3-2). Like the North Star, a code of ethics charts the way for professional behavior and provides a reference point for guidance at difficult junctures.

Librarianship is a profession that prides itself on its ethics of access to information, nondiscrimination, and the right to privacy. These principles are the cornerstones of a librarian's philosophical training. This foundation is crucial in the health information setting, where ethical situations frequently arise in the course of a day's work. We see people trying to circumvent the medical system because they don't trust it, people wanting to use unproven therapies, and young adults researching information that we may think is way beyond their years. As human beings, librarians have feelings and emotions. We cannot, however, let our personal feelings or emotions cloud our professional judgment or influence the scope, level, or depth of health information services we provide or to whom we provide such services.

The reality is that we must apply these codes of ethics to the best of our ability given the scope of our professional practice. It behooves us to become familiar and comfortable with our professional ethics because they provide solid footing in the health information setting.

Moral or Religious Conflicts

As sure as the sun rises and sets, if you're a health information professional for more than a day, you will find your personal morals tested and your ability to keep your personal and religious views to yourself strained. In such a situation, what is your obligation to help? Our professional ethics demand that you put your personal convictions aside and assist the patron. But how does this play out in the real world?

Suppose you have a strong religious belief and someone requests information that goes against its teachings. If you work in a large library with several health reference staff members, you may have a policy whereby a librarian with strong religious beliefs can hand such a patron off to another staff member whose faith would not be affronted by dealing with the question at hand. However, if you are the only staff member on duty or you are a solo librarian, the higher professional ethics of service and intellectual freedom apply. You must put your faith and feelings on the back burner and assist the patron.

> *Everyone on the library staff knows Ann is a staunch Catholic. She attends morning mass daily and observes all the holy days, even coming to work with the ashes on her forehead on Ash Wednesday. Ann works for Regis hospital, a large teaching hospital in a big city. She appreciates the hospital's policy on "Employee Refusal to Care for a Patient Due to Cultural Values, Ethics, or Religious Belief." Ann is working the reference desk at the busy hospital library when an older woman, who looks to be middle-aged, approaches her. She appears nervous and fidgety and*

won't look at Ann. When Ann says, "What may I help you with?" The woman, looking down at her shoes, says in a whisper, "I'm, well, I'm—I'm just trying to find information on, it's um, information on terminating a pregnancy . . ." Ann nods her head and replies, "I'm going to get my coworker, Ingrid, who is really more adept at finding this information. She'll be able to help you find what you're looking for. Just one moment, please."

Note that institutional policies with regard to dispensing information may apply. For instance, if the above interaction happened in a Catholic teaching hospital, Ingrid's reply might have been,

"I'm so sorry. Our hospital policy forbids me to share information on pregnancy termination, but the City of Regis Public Library will certainly be able to help you."

If you will be enforcing a policy whereby librarians may excuse themselves for religious reasons, make sure you practice doing so by role-playing at staff meetings. When the time comes to utilize the policy, you want your staff to be comfortable with the language they'll use, so that their words flow easily and their demeanor is unfazed. You want the transfer from one staff member to another to be seamless and natural, so the patron is not disturbed.

Another moral dilemma librarians face is assisting the patron whose intended use of the information gathered may be for illegal purposes. The salient point here is that *reading material about an illegal activity* is not illegal. The librarian provides reading material across various forms of media—print and nonprint. Assisting a patron in locating information about growing marijuana for medicinal purposes, for example, is not illegal. If the patron goes home and grows marijuana in a state where a medical marijuana law does not exist, then the patron has committed an illegal activity. As difficult as it may be to serve some clients' information needs, our code of ethics supports intellectual freedom and opposes censorship.

On the other hand, *illegal activity in the library* is never condoned. To do so would make you an accomplice to a crime. If you are aware of illegal activity taking place in your library, such as a patron making a drug sale to another patron in the book stacks, report it immediately to security (if you have security services on-site) and call the local police.

Personal Feelings and Emotions

Because librarians are people, sometimes an information request will elicit an unexpected emotional reaction. Each of us brings our life history, good and bad, with us to work. As patrons share their personal stories, we may find we are touched in ways we didn't anticipate and for reasons that are known only to us. We may get teary-eyed or choked up. We may want to laugh inappropriately. Of course, such a response will only trouble our patron. How do we maintain our professional composure given our human nature?

In a library setting with more than one staff member, allow the librarian who is having an emotional response to excuse herself and hand the patron over to another staff person. For instance: "Marie is really our expert on your request, so if you don't mind, I'll ask her to step in."

In such a situation, if you are the only librarian on duty, you may excuse yourself briefly, pull yourself together as quickly as possible, and then return to help the patron. For example: "I can help you with that, but will you excuse me for a moment while I use the restroom?" Then go and run cold water over your face or whatever you need to do to pull yourself together. To stifle the urge to laugh, bite the insides of your cheeks or think unhappy thoughts. The higher ethic of providing access to information and service applies and you must regroup, return, and respond in a professional manner.

If you are visibly upset and unable to excuse yourself before the patron notices, simply be honest. Your show of emotion may actually be touching to your patron. You might say, "I certainly can help you, but right now, as you can see, I'm so moved by your situation that it brought tears to my eyes. I'm so sorry if I've upset you. I imagine this is incredibly hard for you—is there anything I can get for you?" Should you have such a public display of emotion while you are working, be gracious with your patron and gentle with yourself. Keep in mind that you are human and you are dealing with humanity. As you become more experienced in handling requests that push your emotional buttons, you will learn the art of compassionate neutrality—the ability to empathize while keeping your emotions in check.

> *Alice is a new reference librarian who is working alone at Middleton Hospital's Women's Health Resource Center. She is approached by a young woman who says, "Can you please help me?"*
>
> *"Yes, of course; I'd be happy to," replies Alice. "What is it you are looking for?" With a furrowed brow, the woman states, "I'm hoping to find some information on something called AS or happy puppet syndrome."*
>
> *Alice looks at her quizzically. She's never heard of happy puppet syndrome. She imagines in her mind's eye a child with puppet strings dancing merrily along. Alice suddenly wants to laugh. She looks at the woman's face and sees the torment, but she's finding it difficult to suppress her urge. She bites the inside of her cheeks long and hard. Then she says seriously, "Yes, I can help you. Would you first excuse me for just a moment, please?" Alice walks into her office and grabs her face hard, telling herself it's not funny. She talks to herself fast and furiously to pull herself together, realizing that laughter is not so far removed from tears. AS, or Angelman syndrome, is indeed a sad diagnosis of a serious movement disorder. Alice recognizes her response was inappropriate. Returning to the woman, Alice says, "Thanks for giving me a*

moment—I had a program running on my office PC that I needed to close down. Now, let's get started on your request."

Personal Opinions

As a health information professional, it is inappropriate to offer your personal opinion on treatment methods, diagnostic techniques, or healthcare providers. Furthermore, it is inappropriate to share your own personal experiences within the healthcare system with your patrons. Ethically, the health reference encounter is not about you. Perhaps you feel that sharing your experience will be helpful or supportive, but in truth it is merely self-indulgent. As a health information specialist, your personal medical encounters, decisions, treatment regimens, and outcomes are irrelevant. There are legal ramifications for such sharing and these will be discussed more thoroughly in Chapter 4. Suffice it to say, in terms of librarian ethics, this sharing is wrong.

Jill is staffing the consumer health library when a cute young man in blue jeans and a ski jacket approaches her. He is sniffling and tries to suppress a cough, then he says, "I've been looking up L-lysine for canker sores on the Internet and it seems like it might be a good thing to try. I've got a canker sore and it hurts like heck—I mean it's hard to eat anything or even talk and my girlfriend won't kiss me. Have you ever tried this L-lysine stuff? What do think—does it really work? I need to know."

Jill has tried it before and actually swears by it. Yet she cannot respond with, "You'll be glad you looked up that information—it works like a charm for me." Instead she says, "It sounds like you want evidence-based information on the effectiveness of L-lysine in healing canker sores. Let's see what we can find."

Privacy and Confidentiality

Privacy and confidentiality are cornerstones of library service. Since the ALA's first Code of Ethics in 1939 (American Library Association, 1939), they have been a formal part of a librarian's principles of conduct. Librarians may further be governed by state and federal laws, such as HIPAA, the Health Insurance Portability and Accountability Act, to uphold privacy in the workplace. Other federal legislation, such as the Patriot Act, also affects patrons' privacy as well as the way librarians conduct library business (American Library Association, 2002).

The Patriot Act allows law enforcement to obtain a search warrant or subpoena for library items such as books, computer hard drives, patron circulation records, patron Internet access, and so forth, without showing probable cause—the existence of facts to support a belief that a crime has been committed or that said items are evidence of a crime. Under provisions of the Patriot Act, librarians may not disclose that a search warrant was issued *or exists* or that records were produced in compliance. Furthermore, librarians may not inform a patron that library records were shared under the Patriot Act or that an individual is under surveillance by law enforcement officials. In order to uphold the librarian's professional ethic of maintaining patron privacy, review your library policies and procedures to eliminate any unnecessary gathering of your patron's personally identifiable information. For example, look at your library card registration data. What information are you gathering and why? If the answer is, "Because we've always done it that way," that's not good enough. The patron information collected must have a meaningful purpose; otherwise, don't collect it. Similarly, review your current library records retention policy and avoid retaining needless records. Librarians are notorious "keepers." Keeping useless personally identifiable patron information "out of habit" is irresponsible given that we practice librarianship in an era of both increased homeland security measures and identity theft.

Protecting our patrons' privacy means holding confidential any personal information we may come to know while working as librarians. This obligation extends throughout our career and afterward into retirement. Again, our patron's right to privacy is based on state and federal law and our profession's code(s) of conduct. We must guard our patrons' privacy and shelter it as if it were our own. In truth, revealing private information about others can have far-reaching and devastating effects. As we so often see in today's media-frenzied world, the lack of privacy can destroy lives. On a more practical level, it may make us—as well as our employer—vulnerable to a lawsuit.

The necessity of protecting patron privacy extends outside the walls of your library or institution. As a librarian, you may not divulge during your personal time off or away from work what you have come to know professionally about any individual. In providing consumer health information, nothing will kill your business—or your employment—faster than word getting out on the street or throughout your community that you are a gossip or are disclosing your patrons' private information.

The health reference relationship is built on trust, making the protection of privacy paramount—so much so that you may want to advertise, "Our staff keeps your information requests private."

Big cities have an air of privacy about them, but if you are a librarian in a small town, you'll want to make a point of telling your library patrons about your privacy policy. Be sure to point out, "This policy extends outside of the workplace, so if I see you around town, I won't mention your visit. If you want to talk with me about it, you'll need to initiate the conversation."

> *Melissa is tired after a busy day at the Grass Valley Consumer Health Library. She picks up her 10-year-old son from day care and drives him to his soccer game. While sitting on the sidelines relaxing, she sees Abby Miller, a mom of one of her son's teammates, approaching. Abby was in the Consumer Health Library earlier in the day looking up information on*

type 2 diabetes. She puts her lawn chair down next to Melissa and sits. Melissa, respecting Abby's right to privacy, makes no mention of her earlier visit to the library. Instead, she says, "Hey, Abby! Is Aiden as excited about today's game as Zach?"

Serving Children and Youth

Children and youth may be health information seekers, particularly those who have received a medical diagnosis. They may also need information to help cope with a parent's or grandparent's illness. The ALA Code of Ethics, as well as its Library Bill of Rights, included at the end of this chapter (Appendix 3-3), advocates strongly for providing library services to children and youth in any library setting. In the consumer health library, this may take the form of having a well-maintained collection of age-appropriate resources on different health and medical topics. Maintaining a list of appropriate links to authoritative child and youth health Web sites is also suggested. There is further discussion of serving children and youth in Chapter 5.

Serving Mentally Ill or Mentally Challenged Individuals

Anyone who is ill or on medication may exhibit strange behavior; however, strange behavior on the part of someone with a mental illness has a frightening connotation because mental illness still carries a stigma in our country. The truth is, it is often impossible to tell the difference between someone acting out as a result of the stress, physiology, or treatment of a medical diagnosis and someone acting out because of an untreated mental illness or because they are mentally challenged. Ethically, librarians are bound to serve *all patrons* to the best of their ability and without judgment. The benchmark of ideal library service is service that is personalized to the individual's information need in language the person can comprehend. Regardless of whether patrons are having comprehension difficulties because of chemotherapy, Down syndrome, traumatic brain injury, or schizophrenia, our professional ethics require that we strive to meet their information needs with material they can understand. We may do so through a Web site, an interactive tutorial, a DVD or audio CD program, a brochure or fact sheet, a referral to a self-help or support group, or more simply, a book. We choose the most appropriate medium based on our interactions with individuals through conversations or reference interviews that are rooted in our deep respect for others. Further discussion of serving patrons with mental health disorders can be found in Chapter 5.

Summary

As consumer health librarians, our daily interactions with our library users are bound to both delight and challenge us. In challenging times, returning to our Code of Ethics grounds us professionally and reminds us of all we hold dear and aspire to uphold. The ethical practice of librarianship calls for us to:

- put our personal convictions aside and serve the patron,

- promote intellectual freedom and oppose censorship,

- practice compassionate neutrality and keep our emotions in check,

- keep our personal opinions to ourselves,

- protect our patrons' privacy and confidentiality, and

- serve diverse populations with appropriate information.

As we practice delivering health information ethically in the workplace, we ensure that the unique needs of individual patrons will be met with dignity and respect. Since many of us entered the library profession to be of service to others, ethical behavior is an integral part of our philosophical training and daily practice. We are human beings serving humanity to the best of our ability in the health information setting.

References

American Library Association, 1939. Code of Ethics for Librarians. American Library Association. Available: http://www.ala.org/Template.cfm?Section=coehistory&Template=/ContentManagement/ContentDisplay.cfm&ContentID=8875.

American Library Association, 1995. Code of Ethics of the American Library Association. ALA Council. Available: http://www.ala.org/ala/oif/statementspols/codeofethics/codeethics.htm.

American Library Association, 2002. The USA Patriot Act in the Library. American Library Association, Office of Intellectual Freedom. (April). Available: http://www.ala.org/ala/oif/ifissues/usapatriotactlibrary.htm.

Medical Library Association, 1994. Code of Ethics for Health Sciences Libraries. Goals and Principles for Ethical Conduct. Medical Library Association. Available: http://mlanet.org/about/ethics.html.

Appendix 3-1

Medical Library Association Code of Ethics for Health Sciences Librarianship

Goals and Principles for Ethical Conduct

The health sciences librarian believes that knowledge is the sine qua non of informed decisions in health care, education, and research, and the health sciences librarian serves society, clients, and the institution by working to ensure that informed decisions can be made.

Society

- The health sciences librarian promotes access to health information for all and creates and maintains conditions of freedom of inquiry, thought, and expression that facilitate informed health care decisions.

Clients

- The health sciences librarian works without prejudice to meet the client's information needs.

- The health sciences librarian respects the privacy of clients and protects the confidentiality of the client relationship.

- The health sciences librarian ensures that the best available information is provided to the client.

Institution

- The health sciences librarian provides leadership and expertise in the design, development, and ethical management of knowledge-based information systems that meet the information needs and obligations of the institution.

Profession

- The health sciences librarian advances and upholds the philosophy and ideals of the profession.

- The health sciences librarian advocates and advances the knowledge and standards of the profession.

- The health sciences librarian conducts all professional relationships with courtesy and respect.

- The health sciences librarian maintains high standards of professional integrity.

Self

- The health sciences librarian assumes personal responsibility for developing and maintaining professional excellence.

© 1994 Medical Library Association. Used with permission.

Appendix 3-2

Code of Ethics of the American Library Association

As members of the American Library Association, we recognize the importance of codifying and making known to the profession and to the general public the ethical principles that guide the work of librarians, other professionals providing information services, library trustees, and library staffs.

Ethical dilemmas occur when values are in conflict. The American Library Association Code of Ethics states the values to which we are committed, and embodies the ethical responsibilities of the profession in this changing information environment.

We significantly influence or control the selection, organization, preservation, and dissemination of information. In a political system grounded in an informed citizenry, we are members of a profession explicitly committed to intellectual freedom and the freedom of access to information. We have a special obligation to ensure the free flow of information and ideas to present and future generations.

The principles of this Code are expressed in broad statements to guide ethical decision making. These statements provide a framework; they cannot and do not dictate conduct to cover particular situations.

I. We provide the highest level of service to all library users through appropriate and usefully organized resources; equitable service policies; equitable access; and accurate, unbiased, and courteous responses to all requests.

II. We uphold the principles of intellectual freedom and resist all efforts to censor library resources.

III. We protect each library user's right to privacy and confidentiality with respect to information sought or received and resources consulted, borrowed, acquired or transmitted.

IV. We recognize and respect intellectual property rights.

V. We treat co-workers and other colleagues with respect, fairness and good faith, and advocate conditions of employment that safeguard the rights and welfare of all employees of our institutions.

VI. We do not advance private interests at the expense of library users, colleagues, or our employing institutions.

VII. We distinguish between our personal convictions and professional duties and do not allow our personal beliefs to interfere with fair representation of the aims of our institutions or the provision of access to their information resources.

VIII. We strive for excellence in the profession by maintaining and enhancing our own knowledge and skills, by encouraging the professional development of co-workers, and by fostering the aspirations of potential members of the profession.

Adopted June 28, 1995, by the ALA Council Copyright ALA. Used with permission.

Appendix 3-3

Library Bill of Rights

The American Library Association affirms that all libraries are forums for information and ideas, and that the following basic policies should guide their services.

I. Books and other library resources should be provided for the interest, information, and enlightenment of all people of the community the library serves. Materials should not be excluded because of the origin, background, or views of those contributing to their creation.

II. Libraries should provide materials and information presenting all points of view on current and historical issues. Materials should not be proscribed or removed because of partisan or doctrinal disapproval.

III. Libraries should challenge censorship in the fulfillment of their responsibility to provide information and enlightenment.

IV. Libraries should cooperate with all persons and groups concerned with resisting abridgment of free expression and free access to ideas.

V. A person's right to use a library should not be denied or abridged because of origin, age, background, or views.

VI. Libraries which make exhibit spaces and meeting rooms available to the public they serve should make such facilities available on an equitable basis, regardless of the beliefs or affiliations of individuals or groups requesting their use.

Adopted June 18, 1948, by the ALA Council; amended February 2, 1961; amended June 28, 1967; amended January 23, 1980; inclusion of "age" reaffirmed January 24, 1996. Reprinted with permission of the American Library Association.

Chapter 4

Legal Issues in Health Information Delivery

A great deal of mystique surrounds the legal aspects of providing health information to consumers. Some librarians never give it a thought. Others live in fear of patron lawsuits—imagining ruined careers and reputations, not to mention the pain and suffering they may have caused another person. In actuality, patron lawsuits involving the provision of health information by librarians are rare occurrences. In fact, lawsuits are more likely to be brought against libraries and librarians by disgruntled library employees or to involve complex issues such as copyright infringement and Internet filtering protection.

Practicing Medicine without a License

The fact that lawsuits are not common doesn't mean that anything goes. In fact, the potential exists for a lawsuit on several fronts. However, the ethical practice of librarianship is key to averting legal problems. Let's start with the most seemingly innocent offense: sharing your personal opinion on treatment methods, diagnostic tests, or healthcare providers, or sharing the intimate details of your own personal healthcare experience—either with a medical diagnosis or condition, or dealing with the complexities of today's healthcare system. Many librarians think they are being "helpful" by doing so. However, in a legal sense, a tort (or injury) may occur. If anything you say sways or alters the decision making of an individual regarding his or her medical care and the individual suffers as a result, you may violate state business and professional codes. In other words, it may be construed in a court of law that you have practiced medicine without a license. This type of lawsuit is more likely to occur under civil law where fraud and misrepresentation are part of tort law or injury law (Charney, 1978).

How might this work? Let's say you're at the reference desk. You help a patron look up information on a medication for Crohn's disease. The patron says, "I don't understand this." You think you are doing a good job in assisting the patron because you proceed to explain it and embellish your explanation with your own anecdotal experience of the disease. The individual thinks he understands what you told him regarding Crohn's disease and the medication. He follows *your* instructions and, unfortunately, is harmed. Several weeks later you are named in a fraud and misrepresentation lawsuit—practicing medicine without a license. The caveat: it is outside the scope of practice for consumer health librarians to interpret, advise, recommend, or give their personal opinion about the content of the information shared with a patron. As mentioned in Chapter 3, the reference transaction must never be about you. It requires professional practice—interacting with compassionate neutrality.

In the real world of consumer health librarianship, not a day goes by without someone saying, "I don't understand this—can you help me?" To respond appropriately, clarify with the patron exactly what information they are having difficulty with: just one section or an entire piece? Perhaps you are very familiar with the material and could explain it backward and forward. However, in your capacity as a librarian, you must refrain. Instead, offer to find something easier for the person to understand. Consider changing the delivery format of the information (from print to DVD or to interactive Web tutorial). You may also offer a lay medical dictionary. If a patron presses you to "*come on*, just explain it to me," let them know it's outside the scope of your professional practice. You might say something like, "I'm sorry, but by law, I cannot interpret or explain the information to you. However, if you share this information with your doctor or healthcare provider, he or she can explain it to you."

Defamation of Character

Because consumer health librarians are typically considered to be inside the medical establishment, patrons often ask our opinion about a physician's character or skills, or inquire about a medical practice or the reputation of an institution. This is another area that is legally off-limits for you *both on and off the job*. Do not offer opinions, statements, or judgments about a physician's training, reputation, skill set, procedure success rate, and so on. Furthermore, do not offer an opinion on the quality of care or the reputation of a medical practice or medical institution. By doing so, you may open yourself up to a defamation of character lawsuit (Charney, 1978).

> It's a beautiful day and Julia is at the park with her two-year-old daughter. Julia works at Linden Valley Medical Center Library as their consumer health librarian. While Julia is watching her daughter scamper on the park's toddler play structure, Melinda Willis, a daycare provider, approaches her and says, "Hi, Julia. I know you work at Linden Valley and I was just wondering what you think of Dr. Griffin. Is he a good surgeon? Would you trust him? I need to see a surgeon and just don't know who to pick. I hear he has a good reputation. What do you know about him?"
>
> "Well," Julia replies. "I think you'd better keep looking. He's terrible. I just know he has a very bad bedside manner. He's very gruff and he doesn't appreciate his patients asking a lot of questions. Who wants a doctor like that?"
>
> Julia doesn't realize that Miriam Griffin, Dr. Griffin's wife, is sitting nearby watching her three-year-old play and overhears Julia's comments. Of

> *course, Miriam goes home and tells her husband,*
> *"You'll never believe what I heard at the park today!"*
> *It isn't long before Julia is served with court papers*
> *naming her in a defamation of character lawsuit.*

Individuals facing a health crisis want to believe they are getting the best, most effective care. Typically, patrons who ask your opinion about a physician's qualifications or the reputation of a healthcare facility are seeking reassurance. You can respond professionally to such inquiries by stating, "I'm sorry, I can't give you a personal opinion about this particular doctor, but I can help you locate factual information regarding his medical training and board certification. We also have information on how to be an advocate for yourself in the healthcare setting, as well as effective communication tips for talking with your doctor. Would any of these things be helpful to you?" Most patrons are pleased by such a response. For the rare patron who is upset— "What kind of conspiracy is this? I want to know what you *think!*"—you can share the fact that, by law, you cannot endorse or recommend a physician or healthcare facility, but you can share information or help the person locate resources that speak to his or her concerns.

Regarding questions about the reputation of healthcare facilities, there are a number of credible Web sites that offer quality assurance data to patients and the public. The U.S. Department of Health and Human Services offers Hospital Compare (www.hospitalcompare.hhs.gov), an online tool providing comparative information on how well the hospitals in an individual's geographic area care for adult patients with specific *medical* conditions.

The Agency for Healthcare Research and Quality (U.S. Department of Health and Human Services) also has a content-rich Web site (www.ahrq.gov) including, among other features, HCUPnet (part of the Healthcare Cost and Utilization Project), which offers access to health statistics and information on hospital stays at the national, regional, and state level; the Consumer Assessment of Healthcare Providers and Systems (CAHPS) program, which develops and supports the use of standardized surveys that report on and evaluate patients' experiences with healthcare; the National Quality Measures Clearinghouse (NQMC), which is a public repository for evidence-based quality measures and measure sets; and a number of other patient-friendly tools for being an active healthcare consumer.

State government Web sites (e.g., Oregon—www.oregon.gov/ DAS/OHPPR/HQ/ and New York—www.myhealthfinder.com/ newyork06/glancechoose.php) are beginning to post hospital quality indicators for certain medical procedures and diagnoses, comparing outcomes across the state's hospitals. This trend is expected to grow as: (1) consumers are demanding quality care for their valuable healthcare dollars, and (2) the federal government as well as hospital accreditation agencies are placing an emphasis on patient safety and mandating that comparative outcomes data be made available to the public.

The Constitutional Right to Know

Because consumer health librarians practice under ethical and legal constraints, it is important to point out that a librarian's refusal to provide or attempt to restrict information may be found as a violation of an individual's constitutional right to know (Charney, 1978). If a person asks for specific information, you must provide it, given you have it in your collection or possess the skills and resources to access it. In other words, given the capacity to answer, we cannot censure our response to a request for specific information. A minor asking for information about birth control, an elderly patron seeking information about physician-assisted suicide (legal in Oregon), someone who appears depressed wanting information about suicide, a mentally challenged patron asking for information about incest—all of these requests may challenge our personal sensitivities. However, we must not censure these individuals' right to access information if we have it in our library collection or we have the ability to access the requested information given our skills coupled with the library's resources.

Safeguards for Professional Practice

No cases of successful legal action against librarians for providing consumer health information surfaced after an exhaustive search of several EBSCO electronic databases (*Library, Information Science & Technology Abstracts; Health Source: Nursing/Academic Edition; Health Source: Consumer Edition; MEDLINE; Psychology & Behavioral Sciences Collection; Academic Search Premier; Business Source Premier and Professional Development Collection*). However, it is important to keep in mind the "black box" effect. The black box effect in database searching is the inability to see what you haven't retrieved. The fear of being sued survives because we live in a litigious society and the potential exists for the provision of health information to cause harm or injury to the library patron.

To safeguard your practice, a disclaimer statement is recommended. The use of a disclaimer statement regarding the content of the material selected and available to users of your consumer health library, regardless of its format, is meant to protect you, your library, your employees, and your volunteers. A disclaimer is a legal declaration renouncing one's right or claim of responsibility or connection to the actual content of materials in the collection. Prominently display your disclaimer so library users will notice and read it. Tuck a disclaimer statement in materials you send to individuals, including one for mediated searches of electronic databases. You may even want to make a "disclaimer stamp" if you frequently provide such services. A disclaimer will not protect you from legal action, but it does serve as notice to library users that you claim no responsibility for the information presented as fact within the library's resources. In drafting a disclaimer, you may want to garner help from your institution's legal department. See the examples in Exhibit 4-1, Sample Disclaimers.

Tips for Clear Communication

Clear communication is another valuable safeguard for consumer health information professionals. Clear communication consists

Exhibit 4-1. Sample Disclaimers

Consumer Health

1. "All material in the Blakemore Consumer Health Library is provided for information only and should not be construed as medical advice, instruction, or endorsement."

2. "The purpose of the Tulip Valley Medical Center Consumer Health Library is to provide patients and the public with access to a wide range of health and medical information. Our aim is to promote individual responsibility for health and not to offer medical advice. Materials in the library do not necessarily imply any approval or recommendation by Tulip Valley Medical Center Consumer Health Library."

3. "The materials in the Williams Bay Consumer Health Library are intended to provide you with comprehensive information. You may find material that contains information that is different in opinion from that of your physician or healthcare provider. Should any questions arise, please consult with your physician or healthcare provider for clarification about how this information may or may not apply to your unique clinical situation or overall health."

4. "The information in the Alan Sparrow Consumer Health Library is not intended to substitute for medical advice or care from a physician or other healthcare professional. This information is intended for personal use only and is not an endorsement or referral. Please consult your healthcare provider with specific questions."

(Cont'd.)

Exhibit 4-1 *(Continued)*

Mediated Electronic Database Searches

1. "Shepherd Valley Health Resource Center does not assume liability for the accuracy of information or data obtained from third parties, whether in machine-readable or printed form."

2. "When using machine-readable equipment, including computers, be advised that the search results are limited by the databases or Web sites searched, the search engines used, and the searcher's logic and experience."

3. "While every effort is made to ensure the accuracy of information provided, Vista Health Resource Center makes no warranties or representations regarding the accuracy or completeness thereof, and the Vista Health Resource Center disclaims any liability for any damages in connection with the use of its print or electronic resources or services."

of body language and words that are congruent. It leaves no guessing as to the meaning or intent of what is conveyed. Clear communication is straightforward and grounded in the professional ethics and legal parameters that govern all professional librarian interactions. The following tips are important for clear communication.

Things Not to Do

- **Do not** recommend a method or procedure of treatment to follow. For example, *do not* say, "Today, most women with breast cancer have a lumpectomy rather than a mastectomy."

- **Do not** recommend an alternate drug or drugs that may produce the same results as one presently being taken. For example, *do not* say, "Aspirin works just as well as Coumadin for thinning the blood, and it's a lot cheaper."

- **Do not** assist a patron in self-diagnosis, for example, if a patron shows you a red, scaly rash and asks, "What is this?" or "What could this be?" You may locate resources but do not discuss or interpret how or if the information applies to the person's complaint. It's okay to give the person a skin atlas, but do not help identify which rash it appears to be. *Do* encourage the person to seek a medical opinion. You may want to offer information on free health clinics in the area or refer clients to your public health department. People who self-diagnose may not have the financial resources to see a doctor.

The issue of self-diagnosis comes up frequently in the consumer health information setting. In our current healthcare system, physician visits are many times a last resort for patients, not a first resort, unless the individual's symptoms are excruciatingly painful or otherwise compelling. Most people network with family and friends, and try to figure out how to take care of their health problem on their own. They search the Internet or visit a health library looking for resolution. When they've exhausted that effort and the problem remains, they seek medical treatment. You should *expect* to see people who are trying to self-diagnose and self-treat or self-care. Just continue to practice within your professional scope and you'll be fine.

- **Do not** recommend a source as a "best" source. Keep value judgments out of conversations. For example, *do not* say, "MedMaster has the best and most complete drug information." You may indicate, "Many users seem to find this resource helpful," or "This drug handbook contains evidenced-based information on prescription drugs."

- **Do not** guarantee that the information provided by you or your library is accurate, complete, or up-to-date. Remember the disclaimer statement? You don't want to verbally confirm the merits of the information's contents.

- **Do not** indicate that you have done an exhaustive search or uncovered *all* of the information on a topic. This should come as no surprise to a librarian. There is always more information! *Do* emphasize that you are providing information from published materials (including e-resources) that may contain inaccuracies.

- **Do not** say that this is all the information the individual needs. For example, "You'll learn everything you need to know by reading this handy guide" or "This Web site has everything you need to know about polymyalgia rheumatica."

- **Do not** interpret the information, counsel, or attempt to influence the action or decision-making process of the individual. You may interpret the question in order to refine the information request, but you may not explain or translate the materials that respond to the questions. When asked by a patron, "Will you please explain this to me?" or "Can you tell me what this means?" reply, "I'm so sorry, but by law I cannot interpret the information for you. I can offer you a lay health dictionary, if you think that would be helpful. Would you like me to get that for you?" You may also refer the patron to his or her doctor or healthcare provider for an explanation.

- **Do not** offer your personal opinion about a specific therapy, drug, physician, or healthcare organization or your experience of illness or interaction with the healthcare system. For example, if a patron asks, "Have you ever used St. John's wort for depression?" *Do not* respond, "Why, yes, I have and it works great! I'll show you a Web site on it—it's fantastic!" Instead, use a technique called deflection to return the focus of the question back to the patron: "I can show you an online resource that has information on St. John's wort and other herbal remedies. Would that be helpful?"

- **Do not** misrepresent your skills or abilities as a librarian. You are not a physician, nurse, or other medical clinician, therefore you should not diagnose, treat, or recommend tests, procedures, or therapies.

- **Do not** knowingly provide wrong, false, or out-of-date information through oversight or misunderstanding. Replace outdated print materials with current editions *or* remove these items from the collection. At the very least, use a "patron beware" notice to warn the patron that a book is not the current edition. Your message may read: "Note: This book has been superseded by a more current edition" or, more simply, "Note: This book is not the most current edition."

For e-resources:

- **Do not** represent database retrieval as 100 percent accurate. Explain the black box effect and the limitations of search results to your patrons. Teach your patrons that search results are limited by the search engines used (if searching the Internet), the coverage and scope of electronic databases searched, and the skill and experience of the person conducting the search. For mediated searches, use a disclaimer statement, as discussed earlier.

By following these tips on what not to do, you'll be practicing consumer health information delivery that will not leave you vulnerable to a lawsuit. Now let's turn to some things you *can* do.

Things to Do

- **Do** practice at your best level of performance. Keep your skills polished, attend training sessions, participate in consumer health library listservs and blogs, network with your colleagues, and read the professional literature to keep you abreast of current consumer health trends, issues, and resources.

- **Do** keep your collection current within the scope of your budget. Medical information goes out-of-date quickly in today's fast-paced world where instant access to medical breakthroughs and daily press coverage of research results are the norm. For most areas of your print collection, materials that discuss clinical information should be no more than three years old. Materials in the collection that discuss social or psychological issues, such as coping, personal medical stories, grief, death and dying, caregiving, and stress reduction, to name a few, typically have a longer shelf life.

- **Do** know when to refer. Perhaps the individual's information need is outside the scope of the library's service parameters. Refer your patron to the appropriate organization, agency, or individual.

- **Do** remind users that you are a librarian and not a healthcare provider. When someone presses you for help beyond the scope of a librarian's practice, be honest with this gentle reminder. Most people are understanding.

- **Do** establish good communication with users. The heart of good service begins with clear communication.

Summary

Don't let all the dos and don'ts scare you. In the interest of reassurance, consider the words of Ellen Gartenfeld, founder of one of the first cooperative hospital and public library consumer health information networks in the United States, which still ring true today: "As long as librarians don't pretend to be doctors, there's really no problem for them . . . I don't apply any other cautions . . . we're not providing 'do-it-yourself' medicine; we're supporting people in their interaction with their health professionals" (Berry, 1978: 7).

Fortunately, lawsuits against librarians concerning the daily aspects of providing consumer health information are still more feared than a reality. However, for our own well-being and security, it behooves us to practice our profession in a manner designed to minimize the risk of litigation. This means keeping our opinions about physicians and healthcare facilities to ourselves, providing information in accordance with the patron's constitutional right to know, and safeguarding our practices by providing disclaimers. Clearly understanding the scope of the practice of a consumer health librarian and providing reference service within the appropriate parameters are the best assurances against any potential litigation. Clear communication and compassionate neutrality coupled with solid professional skills will help you provide responsive and responsible consumer health reference service.

References

Berry, John. 1978. Editorial, "Medical Information Taboos." *Library Journal* 103, no. 1: 7.

Charney, Norman. 1978. "Ethical and Legal Questions in Providing Health Information." *California Librarian* 39, no. 1: 25–33.

Chapter 5

Serving the Health Information Needs of Diverse Individuals

Each day in the library setting is a mystery as far as who will come use our collection and services. It's part of the joy of our practice as we begin our day—what will today bring and whom will we serve? Meeting the health information needs of all our users is no small task, given the melting pot that is the United States. We serve a diverse clientele and must be confident that we can attend to their requests regardless of who walks in the door. From individuals with physical and mental disabilities, to children and youth, to people whose native language is not English, to minority groups—all come to us seeking direction on their health journey. More than any resource we can point to, it is our interaction with our diverse users that will tell them much about our true desire and commitment to help. Our ability to respond with respect and truly recognize the dignity of each individual will build a bridge for sharing resources with all who seek to know more about their health.

Serving the Disabled

According to the Surgeon General, one in five people living in the United States has at least *one* disability. This is true across all races and ethnicities and in both rural and urban areas (Office of the Surgeon General, 2005). Of course, you can't always tell who has a disability by the way a person looks. Many people live with hidden disabilities such as hearing loss; illnesses such as congestive heart failure, epilepsy, or multiple sclerosis; or chronic pain due to conditions such as degenerative arthritis. Hidden disabilities may include those individuals with developmental disabilities such as autism or other neurological conditions that are diagnosed in childhood and do not diminish over time.

Health information services play a vital role in helping individuals with disabilities obtain important information to live full and meaningful lives. In order to serve these individuals, we must first connect with them. The Surgeon General offers these helpful tips to normalize our interactions:

- See the whole person, not just the disability.

- Speak directly to the person with a disability, rather than through a third party. If the individual doesn't understand you, repeat what you have said, use other words, or find another way to provide the information.

- Speak with adults as adults, and children as children.

- Ask the person with a disability if he or she would like assistance; don't presume help is needed.

- Be aware of and patient regarding the extra time it might take a person with a disability to speak or act.

- Respect what a person with a disability can do. See the ability in disability.

- Understand that not having access to things others take for granted, such as easy access to library services, can cause more problems than the disability itself.

- Be the person who makes a difference. (Office of the Surgeon General, 2005)

Educating individuals—especially those with an acquired disability—about financial and disability resources is an important part of library service. A Financial Toolkit, available either in print or through links on the library's Web site, will help users connect to practical resources that may make a difference in their lives. See the example Financial Toolkit in Exhibit 5-1. Similarly, providing information about the Americans with Disabilities Act (ADA) will help individuals who may not know they are covered gain important legal protections as they cope with and adjust to a life-altering diagnosis. Exhibit 5-2, Americans with Disabilities Act, gives a general definition of disability that an individual must meet in order to receive protection.

Christine, on reference duty, is approached by a young man who is dressed in torn jeans and a dirty T-shirt. He appears a bit nervous and fidgety. Christine smiles warmly and inquires matter-of-factly, "What brings you to the library today?"

"Oh, I don't know. I guess I have . . . like, I saw my doctor and I was in a car wreck and, you know, I haven't been able to work and it's like, I've been having seizures and the doctor tells me I got epilepsy. But man, like, I need to work. I'm young, right? And I need to work. I don't know what I'm gonna do. Does it last forever?"

"I can see that work is important to you and I understand why this is a big concern. You've been through a lot. Would you like some information on epilepsy caused by brain injury? Also, our staff has prepared this helpful guide on financial information for people who are sick or injured."

As she hands him the guide she says, "You might be particularly interested in the section on ADA or the Americans with Disabilities Act, which covers workers with disabling medical conditions."

"Oh, wow, man! Yeah, thanks," he says. "I'll take that and yeah, what've ya got on this epilepsy thing?"

Exhibit 5-1. Financial Toolkit

Assistive Technology

National AgrAbility Project's Web site: AgrAbility.org
http://cobweb.ecn.purdue.edu/~agenhtml/ABE/
Extension/BNG

Provides access to disability-related information relevant to persons living in agricultural and rural communities.

National Rehabilitation Information Center
www.naric.com

Offers a gateway to disability and rehabilitation-oriented information.

USA Tech Guide, United Spinal Association
http://usatechguide.org/techguide.php

See links and resources section for information about financial aid for assistive technology devices.

Each state and territory in the United States has a technology assistance project that has state-specific, up-to-date information on assistive technology, including funding information. Check your state's Department of Rehabilitation, Department of Education, or Department of Social Services, for example, or perform a generic Internet search using the phrase:

[Your State's Name] Assistive Technology.

Many states also have advocacy agencies to assist and advise people with disabilities. Conduct a generic search using terms such as:

[Your State's name] disability (or disabilities) law or [Your State's Name] disability (or disabilities) advocacy.

(Cont'd.)

Exhibit 5-1 *(Continued)*

Employment

Job Accommodation Network
Phone: 800-526-7234; 877-781-9403 (TTY)
http://jan.wvu.edu

Free consulting service designed to increase the employability of people with disabilities. Updates individuals on ADA and disability legislation. Operates under a contract with the U.S. Department of Labor.

Prescription Drug Assistance

The following programs offer prescription drug assistance to individuals who do not have prescription drug insurance coverage and who qualify financially:

Everyone's Rx
www.everyonesrx.com

Rx Assist Patient Assistance Program Center
www.rxassist.org

Rx Outreach
www.rxoutreach.com

Resource Guides

"Annual Resource Guide: A Compendium of Resources for the Special Needs Community: National Organizations, Associations, Products & Services." Exceptional Parent 37, no. 1 (January 2007). (Includes *The Consumer's Guide to Assistive Technology*). Web site for Exceptional Parent: www.eparent.com.

Low-income Clinics

Access to Health Insurance/Resources for Care
www.ahirc.org/index.html

This program started as a service of The Actors' Fund of America's health insurance resource center. With support and funding from the National Endowment for the Arts and the Commonwealth Fund, it has grown to include resources for the self-employed, low-income workers, the underinsured, the uninsured who require medical care, and many other groups.

(Cont'd.)

Exhibit 5-1 *(Continued)*

State and Local Public Health Departments

Each state and territory in the United States has a public health department typically offering some type of healthcare programs for low-income individuals. Contact your local health department by looking in the telephone directory or by performing a generic Internet search: [Your County's Name] health department.

Low-income Healthcare Clinics

To find additional healthcare clinics offering services to low-income or uninsured individuals in your area, check your telephone directory or perform a generic Internet search: [Your State's Name] healthcare clinics low-income; [Your State's Name] dental clinics low-income.

Serving Children and Youth

In order to serve children's health information needs, you'll need a solid understanding of their developmental stages to effectively interact with them and select age-appropriate resources. Use simple language when talking with young children—avoid jargon, acronyms, and euphemisms. If necessary, level the playing field by kneeling down to make eye contact rather than towering over a child. For older children, don't talk down or use slang. Clear, honest communication is best.

At what age is information appropriate? Developmentally, children under three have a strong need for safety and attachment to their parents. Their limited language and cognitive skills make their need for health information minimal. Since play is an excellent way to communicate with very young children, puppets and board books may be helpful resources for parents whose child is ill or hospitalized. For infection-control purposes, you may need to have items that you can give away to this age group. Your Friends of the Library or Hospital Auxiliary group may be willing to assist you by sponsoring these resources.

Children ages three to six years old are learning language skills. This is the age of magic and make-believe. The child's belief in fantasy colors his or her understanding of illness. Simple storybooks may be used to explain medical procedures and illnesses in ways that are meaningful to the child. Helping the child gain an understanding of his or her illness may alleviate expressed or unexpressed fear. Explaining procedures, tests, and treatments to children in very simple language helps to garner their cooperation.

Exhibit 5-2. Americans with Disabilities Act

The Americans with Disabilities Act does not list medical conditions that meet the definition of disability; rather, it has a definition of disability that an individual must meet. For more information, visit the Job Accommodation Network Web site at: http://www.jan.wvu.edu, which is a free service of the Office of Disability Employment Policy, U.S. Department of Labor.

Medical conditions typically protected by ADA (this list is *not* all-inclusive):

- cancer
- epilepsy
- paralysis
- HIV infection
- AIDS
- debilitating stroke
- some learning disabilities
- lung disease
- heart disease
- muscular dystrophy
- multiple sclerosis
- manic depression
- schizophrenia

School-age children (ages six through twelve) are able to understand cause-and-effect, for example, "If I take this medicine, my fever will go down." They are able to think both concretely and abstractly, especially older children in this age range. It's important for the self-esteem of school-age children that they have an understanding of what is happening to their bodies and are included in discussions about their health and medical care. Providing age-appropriate books, DVDs, and Web sites is recommended.

Teens are greatly concerned with establishing their own identity and are grappling with the normal changes their bodies are going through. Illness may be especially troublesome because it singles out the teen at a time in life when he or she desires most to fit in. Privacy is paramount at this age. Health information services to teens must be clear about privacy protections. Service must also be delivered in an open and nonjudgmental manner. Print, multimedia, and Web site resources are all appropriate.

Every child is a future healthcare consumer and should be treated as such. Many librarians rue the day a child stops at the information desk and asks for help on a school health paper. Embrace these requests for the wonderful learning opportunities they are. As with any health reference transaction, this one is an opportunity to teach a child how to be an intelligent advocate for his or her own self-care. It can provide an opportunity for a rich conversation on how to identify quality health information and the reasons why quality matters. Your receptivity, or lack thereof, will tell the child volumes about the services your library has to offer youth and whether or not the library is a welcoming place.

Of course, parents are partners when a child is ill. Their information needs will be deeper and require special sensitivity to their stressful situation. They may need supportive materials on:

- tips for talking with their child about the illness;

- tips for talking with siblings;

- guidelines for communicating with their child's health-care team;

- methods to help them advocate for their child to obtain needed services within both the healthcare system and the school system;

- techniques for coping with the additional strain of having an ill child; and

- support groups and organizations that will provide comfort, encouragement, and assistance.

Colleen is working the information desk when a woman with a young boy approaches. "How may I help you?" Colleen asks.

"Well," the woman starts. "My dad was recently diagnosed with Alzheimer's. He and my son, Adam (she smiles briefly as she looks down at the boy), are very close. My dad has helped care for Adam since he was a baby. I'm trying to find a way to explain his Alzheimer's to Adam, so I thought maybe you'd have something that could help."

"I believe I do," says Colleen. She turns to Adam and asks, "Adam, would you please tell me how old you are?"

Adam shrugs and says, "I'm eight and in the second grade."

"Well, Adam, I just happen to have a book that may help explain your grandfather's illness to you," Colleen states. "Do you enjoy books?"

"Yeah," Adam replies.

Colleen walks to the shelf, pulls the book, Always My Grandpa: A Story for Children About Alzheimer's Disease *(Scacco, 2006), and hands it to Adam. He starts flipping through the pages. "Would you like to check this out?" she asks Adam.*

"Yes, please," he replies.

His mother nods and says, "Thank you so much!"

Serving Patrons with Mental Health Disorders

People with mental health disorders often are isolated by their illness. Similarly, family members fear the unknown, while struggling with the stigma unjustly attached to mental health disorders. Mental illness is often an invisible problem, yet all too common in our society. Each year, about one in four adults ages 18 and older suffer from a diagnosable mental illness (National Institute of Mental Health, 2008). People with mental illness are often discriminated against in any setting because they may act odd or unusual. The consumer health library offers a safe haven—especially if we practice compassionate neutrality—for people with mental health disorders to research their diagnosis and tap into the wealth of coping and management tools available for self-empowerment.

Compassionate neutrality helps us bring a nonjudgmental approach to our work. This is important when interacting with all clients, not just those whom we suspect of suffering from a mental health disorder. Note that people with mental health disorders, like people with physical disorders, may not process information well or may be on medication that affects their behavior or their ability to concentrate and comprehend.

As librarians, we offer our services and resources to all who want them. We communicate with others respectfully and thoughtfully. Even as we try our best to act within the fundamental tenets of our professional ethics, however, there are times when patron behavior challenges us. This, too, is part of the landscape of our work. Look to Chapter 6 for strategies to help you respond to different types of difficult patrons, including individuals who exhibit behavior that makes you feel uncomfortable.

Briefly, these strategies include: remaining calm, speaking slowly and clearly, keeping your hands in view (and watching where the patron's hands are), and not invading the individual's personal space. In their book, *Guidelines for Library Services for People with Mental Illnesses*, Alter and colleagues remind us of two key points: "(1) unusual behavior does not necessarily mean mental illness, and (2) most people with mental illnesses do not exhibit behaviors that call attention to themselves" (Alter et al., 2007). Having a crisis management policy in place, referred to in Chapter 6 as an acceptable behavior policy, and enforcing such a policy are recommended safeguards in the unlikely event that a patron acts out.

> *Vanessa is staffing the circulation desk when a heavyset, disheveled woman and a tall, scruffy-looking man approach. The woman's hair is wild, the man's hair is uncombed, and both are wearing clothes that are a little tattered and not exactly clean. The woman is very agitated and says in a childlike voice, "Can you help us? Can you help us today?"*
>
> *"Yes," Vanessa replies gently. "I can help you."*
>
> *"Oh, good, you can help us. You said you can help us!" She smiles at the man and then at Vanessa.*
>
> *"What is it you need help with?" asks Vanessa politely.*
>
> *"Well, oh, man, all kinds of things, you know— bipolar, ADHD, antisocial and explosive personality disorder—we just need to know everything we can." The woman fidgets and rocks back and forth on her toes, while the man settles into a nearby chair. "Of course, these are for him, not for me. I don't have any of these."*
>
> *"Well, now that I'm clean and sober, I just want to understand what all these things are and what I can do about them," the man volunteers. "I've been clean and sober a month and it's time I looked into all this. They keep telling me I have all these problems and I don't really know what they are."*
>
> *"How about if we start with bipolar disorder and work from there?" Vanessa suggests. She quickly locates an overview of bipolar disorder and the woman reaches for it. As she's reading, she looks up at the man and says, "Acting-out behavior, like*

many affairs. Look at that. You know who they're talking about? Multiple affairs, huh?"

The man shakes his head, rolls his eyes, and says, "You know, I did spend time in jail for attempted murder, but now I'm out and clean for a month." The woman shoots him a knowing look and he stops talking. Vanessa scans the environment, noticing the man's hands folded in his lap. He is quietly observing while the woman is wringing her hands and appears quite anxious and oblivious to that fact that others can overhear the conversation. Two other librarians, Robin and Kim, overhear part of the discussion and place themselves quietly in the background, ready to come forward if needed.

"We have resources on all of the topics you've mentioned. If you'd like, I can show you which section of the library they are in and you can browse. I can also show you specific Web sites if you are interested," Vanessa offers.

"Well, we're in a hurry because we have an appointment soon," the woman says. "Can you just give us some information we can take with us on all this? We've gotta get going, but we'll come back."

"No problem," Vanessa replies. "I'll quickly print some material for you to take today."

Serving Minority and Culturally Diverse Individuals

As we near the end of the first decade of the twenty-first century, the melting pot that is America continues to brew, changing the texture and the richness of our lives in ways unimaginable a generation ago. According to the U.S. Census Bureau, "Large-scale immigration, primarily from Latin America and Asia, underlies both increased racial and ethnic diversity. In just the last two decades of the [twentieth] century, the Asian and Pacific Islander population tripled, and the Hispanic population more than doubled" (Hobbs and Stoops, 2002). Currently, about 25 percent of our diverse population is made up of blacks, Asians, Pacific Islanders, American Indians, Alaska Natives, and Hispanics; ten percent of these Americans are foreign-born (U.S. Census Bureau, 2002).

In a day's work, we may interact with someone whose first language is not English, or who may have a cultural background with a unique perspective on health and healthcare. It may be daunting for minority users to visit the library in the first place, given the fact that language and lack of cultural perspective may be perceived roadblocks. Since the U.S. Census Bureau (2002) reports that "poverty is a fact of life for every racial and ethnic group," it may be more practical matters, such as lack of transportation, that keep people from visiting the library.

As librarians, we are well aware that it is our responsibility to respond as appropriately as possible to patrons from all walks of life and cultural backgrounds. In this way, we may be a bridge between cultures and a repository of the knowledge individuals need to successfully negotiate their important health decisions and self-care. But what does this mean in practical terms? What are the communication keys we need to unlock the barriers of language and cultural differences?

First, offer a receptive environment. Display pictures, posters, and other resources reflective of your community's diverse populations. Purchase library resources in the primary languages spoken in your community and include multimedia as well as print materials. Make sure the materials are not only language-appropriate but also culturally appropriate—not just a foreign-language dubbing of a mainstream DVD, for example. Check nutritional information resources for cultural sensitivity to ensure that recommended foods are typical of the culture and include items likely to be consumed.

Second, exemplify the universal values of respect, friendliness, courtesy, and genuineness, which are crucial in any communication, and particularly in interactions with individuals from other cultures or patrons with limited English-speaking ability.

As librarians on the front line of service, it's our responsibility to become knowledgeable about the customs and traditions of the people we help. We don't have to be experts, but we should have an understanding of the basics.

For example, speaking loudly with many gestures is considered rude in the Vietnamese culture, as is a wave of the hand inviting someone to follow you (LaBorde, 1996). Greeting someone in his or her native tongue is a welcomed gesture, as is knowing key words such as hello, please, and thank-you. These efforts indicate your interest in and willingness to bridge the cultural divide. Giving patrons choices in materials from media-rich resources to simple fact sheets is important, but keep in mind that some individuals will nod in agreement regardless of how appropriately the resources answer their concerns. As best as you can, convey that it is okay to ask for additional information. One time while traveling, a doorman at a hotel answered my every request with the phrase, "Always my pleasure." I was captivated by this response, as I found it incredibly simple yet open and inviting. With three simple words, this doorman left the impression that you could ask him anything. We, as librarians, must aspire to this same level of service and servitude to reach across cultural differences.

As we do our work, it's important to have a frame of reference for other cultures' views of health and healthcare, which are typically much different from those of allopathic or Western medicine. While U.S. medicine is steeped in a tradition of immediate intervention to fix whatever is wrong as quickly as possible, members of other cultures may adopt a wait-and-see approach and strive to accept their diagnosis with grace and dignity. This different frame of reference may influence the type of information sought and may be more focused on complementary or natural therapies than on conventional approaches.

If you haven't done so, you might consider implementing an educational component at your monthly staff meetings that features the different cultures in your community. There are many online resources available, too, and these are listed in Exhibit 5-3, Multicultural Resources.

Exhibit 5-3. Multicultural Resources

Web Sites

Ethnomed: www.ethnomed.org

Health Information Translations: www.healthinfotranslations.com

Healthy Roads Media: www.healthyroadsmedia.org

RHIN—Refugee Health Information Network: www.rhin.org

Spiral—Selected Patient Information Resources in Asian Languages: http://spiral.tufts.edu

The 24 Languages Project: http://library.med.utah.edu/24languages

Helpful Guides

Clay, Edwin S., III. 2006. "They Don't Look Like Me: Library Multicultural Awareness and Issues." *Virginia Libraries* 52, no. 4 (October–December): 10-14. Available: http://scholar.lib.vt.edu/ejournals/VALib.

IFLANET: International Federation of Library Associations and Institutions. 2002. *Multicultural Communities. Guidelines for Library Services.* 2nd ed. revised. Available: www.ifla.org/VII/s32/pub/guide-e.htm.

An Asian man approaches the information desk. He is dressed in a suit and tie. He makes eye contact briefly with Joyce, the reference librarian on duty, and bows slightly. Joyce bows slightly in return and says, "Welcome. How may I help you?"

The man says in broken English, "Yin cansa, me have."

Joyce nods and points to her chest, "Lung cancer?"

The man shakes his head no. "Yin, yin cansa."

"Oh, skin cancer?" Joyce says while pointing to her arm.

"Yes," the man replies.

"Please, may I ask you, do you speak a language other than English?" Joyce asks.

"Hai, hai," the man says smiling. "Japanese."

"Japanese, very good. Domo arigato," Joyce nods in response. "Now, would you like skin cancer information in English or Japanese?"

"Oh, Japanese, please," he replies. "Thank you. Thank you very much."

"My pleasure," Joyce responds and begins to walk over to a computer. "Please come with me." She pulls up an explanation of skin cancer on the Health Information Translations Web site [www. healthinfotranslations.com] that is written in both English and Japanese.

Serving LGBT Individuals

The exact number of lesbian, gay, bisexual, and transgender individuals in the United States is not known because so many of these individuals are closeted. Even men who have sex exclusively with men may not consider themselves gay (Pathela et al., 2006). A report by the Human Rights Campaign estimates that 5 percent of the total U.S. population ages 18 years and older are lesbian or gay (Smith and Gates, 2001). Understandably, stigma and prejudice keep many LGBT individuals guarded about their sexual identity.

Librarians have a long history of supporting the LGBT community. In 1970, the American Library Association (ALA) formed the Task Force on Gay Liberation, which eventually became a unit of ALA now known as the Gay, Lesbian, Bisexual and Transgendered Round Table (GLBTRT). It was the nation's first gay, lesbian, bisexual, and transgender professional organization (Gay, Lesbian, Bisexual and Transgendered Round Table, 2008). For its part, the Medical Library Association has an LGBT Special Interest Group, established in 1994.

As librarians, we are called to continue honoring this proud history in our daily work. Often, we won't know if someone is lesbian, gay, bisexual, or transgendered. Like any other individuals who come to the library, LGBT people have unique health information needs they want addressed and it is our responsibility to help them with nonjudgmental compassion.

Like most people, LGBT individuals look for environmental clues that communicate a welcoming place. Such clues include brochures and posters about LGBT health concerns, such as ovarian, breast, or cervical cancers, non-Hodgkin's lymphoma, STDs, and safe sex. Posting a visible nondiscrimination statement is also helpful. Displaying the universally recognized LGBT-friendly symbol of the rainbow flag or pink triangle is a clear indication of receptivity.

As for communication tips, simply talk and interact with an LGBT individual as you would any other library user—with openness, empathy, and respect. Encourage trust by explaining that all library transactions are kept confidential. Be mindful of your language and terminology when interacting with LGBT individuals. Follow their lead by using the same descriptive term and pronoun for sexual orientation if they self-identify. Like all minorities, understand that LGBT individuals may be more sensitive or defensive than other patrons because of the level of social discrimination, prejudice, and outright hostility they may have received. Your ability to connect with and support them on

Exhibit 5-4. LGBT Resources

Web Sites

Gay & Lesbian Medical Association (GLMA):
www.glma.org

MedlinePlus: Gay, Lesbian and Transgender Health:
www.nlm.nih.gov/medlineplus/
gaylesbianandtransgenderhealth.html

National Coalition for LGBT Health:
www.lgbthealth.net

Parents, Families and Friends of Lesbians and Gays (PFLAG):
www.pflag.org

Seattle/King County LGBT Health Web Pages:
www.metrokc.gov/health/glbt

Transgender Law Center (TLC) Healthcare Publications:
www.transgenderlawcenter.org/publications.
html#healthcare

Helpful Contacts

GLBT Help Center
888-THE-GNLH (843-4564); www.glnh.org

Offers toll-free peer counseling, information, and local resources.

GLBT National Youth Talkline
800-246-PRIDE (7743)

Peer counseling, information, and local resource referral for youth through age 25.

their health information journey is invaluable. For a list of helpful resources, see Exhibit 5-4, LGBT Resources.

> *Jeanne, a reference librarian in a busy consumer health library, is approached by a young man who appears quite shy. He seems nervous and says haltingly, "Umm . . . I wonder if you could help me. I mean, I don't know if the library can help me or not. But I was wondering if you had anything on . . ."*
> *He pauses here and thinks about it, then continues in a whisper, ". . . uh, coming out?"*
>
> *Jeanne smiles warmly and says, "I'm sure I can help you find some information. Just to clarify, are you wanting information on coming out to your parents or family members?"*
>
> *The young man nods "Yes."*
>
> *"Okay, we have some wonderful Web resources for support," Jeanne says reassuringly. "There may also be a PFLAG group in the area—Parents, Families and Friends of Lesbians and Gays—so let's check that. And of course, we have printed materials, such as books. What would you like to do first?"*
>
> *The young man breathes a sigh of relief and says, "The Web, please!"*

Summary

Serving the health information needs of diverse individuals is all in a day's work for a consumer health librarian. From helping people with physical or mental disabilities, to children and youth, to those with different language or cultural backgrounds, to LGBT individuals, it is all part of the rich texture in the fabric of a typical day. Regardless of whom we serve, we are responsible for communicating effectively. Knowing appropriate communication skills to interact with a wide variety of library users will make our patrons more at ease, allowing us to be more successful in our work. Looking past obvious differences and responding to the heart of each person who seeks our service enables us to interact with sensitivity. We may not always be perfect in our attempt to bridge these differences smoothly, but patrons will forgive our small foibles if they recognize our earnestness. The enduring values of respect and compassion shine through when we are genuine with others.

Additional Reading

Liu, Yi Hui, and Martin T. Stein. "Talking with Children." In: Parker, Steven, Barry Zuckerman, and Marilyn Augustyn, eds. 2005. *Developmental and Behavioral Pediatrics: A Handbook for Primary Care*. 2nd ed. Philadelphia: Lippincott Williams & Wilkins.

References

Alter, Rachel, Linda Walling, Susan Beck, Kathleen Garland, Ardis Hanson, and Walter Metz. 2007. *Guidelines for Library Services for People with Mental Illnesses*. Chicago: Association of Specialized and Cooperative Library Agencies, American Library Association.

Gay, Lesbian, Bisexual and Transgendered Round Table. 2008. American Library Association. Available: www.ala.org/ala/glbtrt/welcomeglbtround.cfm.

Hobbs, Frank, and Nicole Stoops. 2002. *Demographic Trends in the 20th Century*. Census 2000 Special Reports, Series CENSR-4, U.S. Census Bureau. Washington DC: U.S. Government Printing Office.

LaBorde, Pamela. 1996. "Vietnamese Cultural Profile." *EthnoMed*. Available: http://ethnomed.org/ethnomed/cultures/vietnamese/vietnamese_cp.html.

National Institute of Mental Health. 2008. "The Numbers Count: Mental Disorders in America." National Institutes of Mental Health. Available: http://www.nimh.nih.gov/health/publications/the-numbers-count-mental-disorders-in-america.shtml.

Office of the Surgeon General. 2005. "The Surgeon General's Call to Action to Improve the Health and Wellness of Persons with Disabilities." U.S. Department of Health and Human Services, Office of the Surgeon General. Available: www.surgeongeneral.gov/library/disabilities/calltoaction/index.html.

Pathela, Preeti, Anjum Hajat, Julia Schillinger, Susan Blank, Randall Sell, and Farzad Mostashari. 2006. "Discordance between Sexual Behavior and Self-reported Sexual Identity: A Population-based Survey of New York City Men." *Annals of Internal Medicine* 145: 416–425.

Scacco, Linda. 2006. *Always My Grandpa: A Story for Children About Alzheimer's*. Washington, DC: Magination.

Smith, David M., and Gary J. Gates. 2001. *Gay and Lesbian Families in the United States: Same-sex Unmarried Partner Households: A Preliminary Analysis of 2000 United States Census Data. A Human Rights Campaign Report.* (August 22). Washington, DC: Human Rights Campaign. Available: http://www.hrc.org/documents/gayandlesbianfamilies.pdf.

U.S. Census Bureau. 2002. "The Population Profile of the United States: 2000." (Internet Release). Available: www.census.gov/population/www/pop-profile/profile2000.html.

Chapter 6

The Difficult Patron

If only a day in the reference setting went by without having to deal with the dreaded *difficult patron*. They come in all shapes and sizes and sometimes with a new twist on an old theme. In our professional training, few of us were taught how to interact effectively with patrons who pose special challenges. We may stumble and get upset or we may act surprised and stymied when we're caught off guard. Such responses only help to make a bad situation worse. Our desire is to always act professional: cool, calm, and collected under any circumstances. But how do we achieve this when someone insists on pushing our buttons or, worse yet, frightens us? Read on for some helpful strategies!

Unless we are well skilled in communication techniques, when stressed we often resort to automatic responses in our effort to try to regain control of the situation. After all, stress is the perception that things are out of control, and we may feel that we simply don't have the capacity to cope or to handle the situation. We want instant relief, and therefore we act or speak without thinking. You've heard such retorts before: "Because we've always done it that way," or "It simply won't work!" or "We can't," and so forth. These comebacks are typically knee-jerk reactions, not well-thought-out, logical responses. We dig our heels in with such a quick, unthinking reply. Automatic responses put both parties immediately on the defensive. In our attempt to quickly quash the uncomfortable feelings caused by these stressful encounters, we've polarized the issue, which only serves to escalate any tension. Isn't there a better way? Of course there is.

The Four-Step Approach

One way to regain real self-control in tense situations is by using a technique called the Four-Step Approach, as outlined in *The Wellness Book: The Comprehensive Guide to Maintaining Health and Treating Stress-related Illness* (Benson and Stuart, 1992). This four-step approach gives you an opportunity to take a time-out, so to speak, and quickly evaluate the situation before responding. It buys you time to assess the situation and formulate a response in a calm and rational manner. It works like this:

- Step 1, STOP: Cut off the craziness in your mind. Tell yourself to *stop* any anxious thoughts or negative self-talk.

- Step 2, BREATHE: Take a deep breath to release tension and calm yourself. As you read this paragraph, make a fist. That's it, a big fist. Now, as you make this fist, what are you doing with your breath? Most likely, you're holding it. That's what we do when we are under stress—we tense our muscles and literally hold our breath. So, breathe—a nice, deep belly breath. If you were a "choir kid" you know what this means: the kind of breath you inhale deeply through your nose into your diaphragm and then exhale slowly. Please don't sigh; remember from our earlier chapter that sighing is off-putting. No one has to know you are taking this deep, luxurious, calming breath. It's a little gift to yourself.

- Step 3, REFLECT: Ask yourself, what is really going on here? What am I protecting? Do I need to? What will happen if I say "yes" or bend the rules? What will the consequences be? What personal buttons of mine are being pushed? Do I need to distance myself emotionally from this situation in order to handle it responsibly? In reflecting, we are taking a moment to put the situation into perspective, briefly weighing whether our personal feelings are distorting the situation while asking a central question: "How important is this?"

- Step 4, CHOOSE: Choose to respond rather than simply react. Now that you are calm and have more clarity about the situation, communicate that you are willing to find common ground to resolve the situation. "I'd really like to hear what you have to say" or "You're right; how can we work this out?" or "What do you need right now?"

The four-step approach offers us a path to self-control in stressful situations. It gives us time to step back and reassess a situation and our own feelings about it before jumping in and trying to fix it. It helps us to see the bigger picture and respond in a way that is both respectful and rational. You'll find it comes in handy in many difficult patron interactions.

The Angry Patron

You might think as a consumer health librarian that you needn't worry about angry patrons, because patients are never angry, right? *Oh, so wrong!* Patients have all kinds of things to be angry about regarding their healthcare today, for example: the battery of expensive and invasive diagnostic tests they may be undergoing, the length of time it can take to work through the diagnostic process, the high costs of healthcare, the perceived incompetence of their healthcare provider, the frustration of trying to navigate the bureaucratic maze of large healthcare organizations, and so on.

Just where does anger come from? Anger is an emotional response to a perceived injustice or violation. Something hasn't gone right or has been handled poorly. Angry people are not particularly rational because they feel they have been wronged. They are seeking justice; they want their wrong righted. Even though you as a consumer health librarian may have nothing to do with the perceived injustice, you may be the individual who bears the brunt of the patron's anger. Some patients are angry at their illness and you may be seen as a safe target at which to vent this anger. So, what to do?

- Maintain your composure

- Level the playing field

- Defuse the situation

One way to maintain your composure is to use the four-step approach outlined above: Stop-Breathe-Reflect-Choose. As you are going through each of the four steps, be sure you maintain eye contact with the patron. Don't stare or glare, but simply look at the other individual and blink as necessary. Take a deep breath and ground yourself. As you are doing so, listen to what the individual is *really* saying. Is this person truly angry to the point of being dangerous, or is he or she completely frustrated or deeply scared and this is a way of expressing those feelings? Can you hear where the injustice or the perceived wrong occurred?

Luckily for you, because people are not mind readers, the patron will not know you are silently moving through the four-step approach, and that's just fine. As you are quietly breathing and reflecting, the patron may calm down because you are not "fighting back." A most important point in interacting with an angry person is that perhaps more than anything else, he or she simply wants to be *heard* and *understood*.

You level the playing field by moving your body into alignment with the angry patron. If the patron is standing, you stand. If the patron is sitting, you sit down. At the same time, open up your body posture to a nonconfrontational pose. If you are standing face-to-face, bring your body to a more side-by-side stance with the individual. The meaning of your powerful nonverbal body language changes from "We're pitted against each other" to "We're on the same side." Often, an angry patron will begin to lower his or her voice as you move your body into symmetry.

For your personal safety, make sure you know where the individual's hands are at all times. Keep your own hands in front of you where they can be seen by the patron. Remember that open palms send a positive nonverbal message. Watch your personal space as well. If the patron is clearly agitated, keep a leg's distance away. You can still use the open posture stance mentioned earlier; regardless of whether you are close to the individual or a leg's stance away, it still sends the same nonverbal message: "I'm on your side."

Now that you've stopped-breathed-reflected-chosen, you are calmer. Begin trying to peacefully resolve the situation. Look the patron in the eye when you talk. Don't stare, but do make eye contact to maintain a connection. Keep your facial expression as relaxed as possible; this requires self-awareness in a difficult situation. For example, try not to frown or scowl. Ideally, your tone of voice is calm and soothing. When you talk, be sure to talk slowly because angry people cannot process information quickly. In fact, studies indicate that they hear about 7 percent of what you are saying, so keep it simple. Use the active listening technique, where you repeat what the individual just told you in the form of a question. For example, "I hear you say you've had it with your doctors and all the tests. Is that correct?"

These techniques will not come easily unless they are practiced. Use role-playing exercises as part of your staff meetings to give librarians experience in defusing an angry patron. If you are a solo librarian, ask a friend to role-play with you or practice in front of a mirror.

It's important to remember, you *can* interact successfully with an angry patron by maintaining your poise through use of the stop-breathe-reflect-choose technique, putting yourself and your patron on equal footing by leveling the playing field, and calming the situation by communicating clearly with the individual. Remember, most angry people are seeking confirmation. Healthcare is tough these days. A diagnosis or lack of one can make an individual distraught. Losing a loved one or watching a loved one suffer or endure a painful illness may provoke anger. By employing the techniques outlined here, you should be able to calm most patrons.

In the event the individual is not soothed but grows angrier, you must state clearly, "I need you to please calm down or I will call security." You may have to repeat this once, but if there is no evidence the individual is calming down, it's time to call security or follow the security plan for your library. Above all else, protect yourself and other patrons in this situation.

An elderly gentleman enters the library and appears greatly upset. When Esme, the reference librarian, approaches him, she smiles and says, "May I help you?" "You think you're going to help me?" he snaps. "Are these books and computers going to make me well? I have cancer, for goodness' sake. CANCER!"

Moving closer, Esme says gently, "I understand you are upset by your diagnosis. It's agonizing and perhaps frightening. I'm so sorry you are in that uncomfortable place, where you know what's wrong but don't understand it. I'm sure some part of you is curious. Is that what brings you to the library today? What can we do while you are here to help you feel better? Is there anything in particular you want to learn about?"

With that, the gentleman grumbles a bit and then says, "Well, he told me I have non-Hodgkin's lymphoma. I have no idea what this is. I just want to know what this is, what it does to you, how the treatment works."

Esme says, "I can definitely help you with that. We have several options: Would you like to read about it, have me show you the Leukemia & Lymphoma Society's 'newly diagnosed' section of their Web site, watch a DVD, or all of the above?"

"Well, if it isn't too much trouble, all of the above! I need to learn everything I can," replies the gentleman, who now appears much more relaxed.

The Complainer

Do you dread the patron who complains about your policies or service? Is your automatic response to a suggestion, "No!"? Perhaps it isn't the idea of change that upsets you as much as it is the messenger or the way the complaint is delivered. Either way, if you work in a library, or for that matter any workplace, you will at some time have to deal with a complaint. Often, the automatic response to a complaint comes from a defensive posture. We feel we need to defend ourselves or our workplace because we find something in the complaint threatening, and so our automatic response is, "No!" We may unthinkingly pit ourselves against the patron. Again, there is a better way.

The wisest thing you can do to deal successfully with a complaint is to reframe it: change your attitude about it from something negative to something more positive. For example, instead of lamenting, "This complaint is going to waste my valuable time," reframe your attitude to "This complaint is an opportunity to learn something new about our library service."

Use the four-step approach to help you adjust and open up your attitude: stop-breathe-reflect-choose. As you breathe and reflect, move your thoughts from dread at hearing the individual's complaint to being receptive and hearing the concern. A good complaint may help you improve your service or library environment so try to adjust your attitude from an automatic, defensive reaction to one of openness and receptivity. Remember the old business adage, "For every complaint you receive, ten other people are thinking the same thing but are too timid to tell you." This complainer is invested in your library and wants improvement, and is thereby speaking up while other patrons may have given up. This individual is doing you a favor.

When responding to a patron complaint, first acknowledge the person's feelings: "I see you are upset about this. Please tell me about it." Then let the individual explain the problem. Do not interrupt or argue with the person; just let them talk. Make sure you understand the complaint by asking questions to clarify if necessary. Then ask the $64,000 question: "What can we do to correct the situation?" Another valuable question you can ask is, "What do you need?"

Some complaints can be resolved on the spot. If you need to uphold a policy, explain why. For example, "I understand you wanted to spend more time on the computer, but as you can see, we have a group of people waiting for their turn. In fairness to all, our policy is to limit computer access to one-hour sessions. Your understanding and cooperation are much appreciated."

If possible, offer the individual choices to increase his or her sense of control in resolving an unhappy situation. For example, "I understand the book you wanted to check out has a hold on it for another patron, and you're upset that we won't cancel the hold. I'm sure you understand that wouldn't be fair to the individual who is waiting for it. I can put your name next in line for this book. In the meantime, I can check to see if another copy is available or I can help you find a similar book. Would that be helpful?"

Some complaints are more serious and not as easy to resolve, such as a complaint about the appropriateness of a book in your collection. Usually such serious complaints must be put in writing, and having to do so may discourage some patrons. Yet this is good library practice. Requiring written challenges to materials in the collection formalizes the complaint and should set in motion both procedures and documentation for appropriate follow-through and follow-up. It's imperative that you have a complaint policy for your library and that all staff follow the steps outlined when formal complaints are submitted.

Complaints obviously raise questions about library services, hours, policies, and procedures and may encourage long-overdue and necessary change. Reframing complaints from problems to potentials gives you an opportunity to review how you are doing things in your library and why. The key questions include: "Is this still working? Can it be improved? Is it indeed time to update? Is it perhaps time to tighten a procedure or even loosen one up a bit? What is in both the library's and the users' best interests at this point in time? How can we make this work?" Using complaints as learning opportunities ensures that your library will be a vibrant place of information service. Your responsiveness to your users' concerns coupled with your patrons' ability to successfully question library operations reinforces the important relationship you share. Now that's something positive!

Sparrow Consumer Health Library has been successfully serving the patient population of Sparrow Hospital for years. Kathryn Miller is the director and she's very proud of her library. One day, a staff member comes into her office and says, "Kathryn, I have a patron who is unhappy about our book loan period. Will you please come and talk to her?"

Kathryn smiles and says, "Of course." She thinks, "Hmmm . . . I wonder what I'm going to learn today about my library!"

Kathryn approaches the woman and says, "I hear you have something important to say about our book loans. Please tell me what's on your mind."

"Well," the patron says, "I'm Linda Singer and I've been using this library for years. I'm just suggesting that two weeks is really too short a time to borrow a book from this library. I mean, if you're undergoing tests or treatment you can't be running back and forth to the library all the time!"

Kathryn nods her head affirmatively and says, "That's a very valid point. I hadn't thought of it that way. We were trying to make the books available to as many people as possible by having a shorter loan period. You've given me something to think about. What amount of time would you think is reasonable?"

Linda thinks for a minute, and then says, "Well, three weeks would be helpful."

"I really appreciate your bringing this concern to my attention. I'll tell you what; I'll direct the staff to change the loan period on the items you want to borrow today to three weeks. Then I'll discuss your request with the staff at-large and get back to you. It may be time to change our loan policy. Again, thank you for saying something about this."

Linda is thrilled. "Thank you!" she gushes.

Two weeks later, Linda receives a letter from Kathryn Miller stating that the Sparrow Consumer Health Library has changed its book loan period from two weeks to three weeks. Linda is thrilled and tells all of her friends and family what a wonderful place the Sparrow Library is.

The Frequent Flyer

I know you've seen them—the patrons who return repeatedly with the *same unresolved issue or question*. They come in over and over and it's always the exact same question. They take up *a lot* of your time. You're at your wit's end because you've showered them with materials, Web sites, full-text articles from electronic databases, referrals to other agencies in the community, etc., and still, here they are visiting you again (!) with the *same* information need. These are not merely patrons seeking clarification, but patrons who stymie you because you don't see them making any progression on their health information journeys after repeated visits to the library. There is an explanation: you are dealing with "frequent flyers."

Frequent flyers are patrons who receive an abundance of time and attention from you, which is nice, but the fact is, they are not really seeking health information. Frequent flyers are actually venting their displaced frustration on someone who is perceived as a good sounding board: you. These individuals feel victimized by their diagnosis or health dilemma. Sadly, they are trapped by their feelings of powerlessness to effect any real change regarding their health.

Why do they hang around the library and take up so much of your time? It's safe. Frequent flyers view you as someone who is nonthreatening. They are trying very hard to gain some measure of control over a difficult health situation *without actually taking personal responsibility for the outcome*. They want to feel better without having to resolve the difficult choices confronting them, making them literally stuck in their own indecision. You, a consumer health librarian, are not seen as being able to actually help solve the dilemma. Since you don't threaten their status quo, it makes you a safe harbor in their health storm.

Therefore, all of your attempts to find appropriate materials and resources are quickly rejected or explained away. This happens time after time after time. You get to the point where you have truly exhausted your expertise on this same question. It takes time, but eventually you realize you have a frequent flyer before you. Once the realization occurs, what can you do?

Three helpful steps will see you through this difficult patron interaction:

- Disengage

- Use active listening

- Return responsibility

Yes, the first step is to disengage, which is anathema to a librarian's nature. However, this situation calls for it. So stop trying to find more materials, resources, or solutions. Move instead to active listening.

Allow the individual to vent or describe the problem (even though you are already very familiar with it). Paraphrase what you heard described: "I hear your doctor wants you to consider a clinical trial for your type of cancer. Is that correct?" Keep your emotions in neutral. Listen as the person talks and keep paraphrasing back.

Finally, return the responsibility for his or her health back to your patron. Don't be tempted to offer more help through additional materials or resources; as in all the other instances before, they will only be batted away or rejected. It's okay to tell the person you have exhausted your expertise or you are out of ideas. If he or she asks you, "What should I do?" you can respond again by turning the responsibility back to the individual: "Only you can decide in consultation with your doctor."

The interesting thing is, once you disengage, you stop giving the frequent flyers what they seek most—attention and a sense of control. Guess what? They often move on at this point. They'll seek a new sounding board.

Dealing with frequent flyers is difficult and emotionally draining for most consumer health librarians. You see patients who need treatment badly, but cannot bring themselves to consent. They are frozen with fear. You can suggest social services to your frequent flyers, but odds are, they will refuse or tell you, "I tried it and it just didn't work for me."

Frequent flyers can be hard to identify because it takes time to realize what is going on with this particular type of patron interaction. You'll suspect it when you are frustrated by the same patron who repeatedly visits the library with the same information need. This is a most difficult patron to deal with because librarians are taught to provide service, not withhold it. Remind yourself that you *have* provided service over and over again to this individual to no avail. It's time to move forward by disengaging, listening actively, and returning responsibility to the patron.

> *A middle-aged man approaches Jen at the information desk and asks her for information on stage IV prostate cancer clinical trials. Jen helps him search both the National Cancer Institute's Clinical Trial Database (www.cancer.gov/clinicaltrials) and the National Institutes of Health clinical trials Web site (www. clinicaltrials.gov). She spends a great deal of time retrieving information on specific clinical trials and also the nuts and bolts of the clinical trial process.*
>
> *A week later, the same man asks her for the same information. She asks, "Well, I think I remember you; haven't we searched this already?" To which he says, "Not really. That other information wasn't right. I only want clinical trials on stage IV prostate cancer." "Okay," Jen replies. "We'll try again."*
>
> *Two weeks later, he returns. Again, Jen is working. She sees him and wonders to herself, "What's up?" He comes over and says, "You've helped me before. Can you help me again?"*
>
> *"Of course," Jen says.*
>
> *"I have prostate cancer. Stage IV. My doctor thinks I should consider a clinical trial. Can you help me find out what's available?"*
>
> *Jen can't believe it! She thought for sure he would have different concerns. She really doesn't want to do this search yet again. "Yes, I remember helping you before. We've searched for information on the*

specific trials for which you might qualify and also information to help you learn how clinical trials are conducted, what types of trials there are, what expenses may be covered, and so forth. What do you need this time?"

"All of the above!" he says enthusiastically. "That other stuff just didn't get to the point." Although she's feeling frustrated because the patron has already received the information she is retrieving again, she gets to work. She starts to think maybe he's a frequent flyer.

Another two weeks pass and the man returns once more. This time Jen is prepared. He approaches her and, sure enough, asks her for information on stage IV prostate cancer clinical trials.

She listens and says to him, "I understand you have stage IV cancer of the prostate. I know you are looking for clinical trial information. I must tell you that I've exhausted my research capabilities on this request."

"Well, what do you mean? I have cancer! I need clinical trial info!" he declares.

"Yes, yes, I know. You have prostate cancer. You need clinical trial information. I'm really sorry, but I have exhausted my expertise in helping you find relevant material," Jen states.

"Well, then. What should I do? What would you do if you were me?" he wonders aloud.

"I think you know best what you can do. Take the information you have found and your questions to your doctor and talk this over."

"Well, what should I do?" he asks again.

Jen looks him in the eye and says softly, "I think you know best what you can do. Take the information you have found and your questions to your doctor and talk this over."

With that, the man takes his leave.

The Guarded Individual

Some patrons enter the consumer health library and, instead of making their way to the information desk, they turn in the opposite direction and just walk around or browse. They consciously turn away from the staff. These patrons avoid eye contact and their body language is pulled inward. These individuals may be considered guarded patrons—people who are literally "on guard." Guarded patrons are usually silent and uncommunicative. They won't seek you out. They come to the library because they have competing needs: a desire to know and understand their diagnosis vs. a fear of what they may learn.

Often, guarded patrons are afraid or anxious. They're hesitant to share their information need. What is most important to these individuals? Privacy.

So, how might you help this type of patron? In a nutshell: gently. When approaching a patron who is guarded, use a soft, calm voice. Avoid an abrupt or businesslike tone because these individuals are already anxious and you want your approach to be nonthreatening. Ease them into conversation by making small talk about commonalities such as the weather or a local sports team. When you are ready to move into the nature of their library visit, use open-ended questions to engage them in dialogue. For example, use open-ended questions such as "How may I help you today?" or "What brings you to the library today?" rather than the dead-end, closed questions "Do you need help?" or "Can I help you?"

Give the individual time to respond. Guarded individuals are not going to win any reference races, so slow down and don't hurry or try to rush them along. Employ body language that facilitates trust. For example, open up your stance—the side-by-side stance is important here ("I'm on your side"), lean in slightly toward the individual, and have your arms down at your sides with your palms facing up. As you conduct your reference interaction, look the individual in the eye and maintain a warm, welcoming facial expression.

Sometimes guarded individuals won't share their information needs; this is okay. It's always a good idea to reaffirm the library's privacy policy for these individuals and then simply offer to show them how to conduct a generic search. Keep your explanations as matter-of-fact as possible. You could say, "I thought you might like to know that all visits to the Smith Consumer Health Library are confidential and we protect our patrons' privacy. Now, I'd like to show you how to find information on, let's say, arthritis. It's very simple and once you know what steps to follow, you'll be able to find information on any topic all by yourself!" Once guarded individuals learn they can trust you, they will be more likely to seek your assistance.

Of course, you must respect a guarded individual's right not to be helped. Some people will come into the library three or four times and refuse assistance. They may be fighting an inner battle: "I want to know about my disease, but I'm afraid of knowing about it." Give them time. Continue to be warm and receptive. The guarded individual will ultimately make a choice and when they are ready to delve into learning, they will have observed and thereby know you are available to help them on their journey.

> *It's a cold winter day and a woman walks into the library and glances around. She walks along the periphery of the library, just noticing the books, magazines, and computer stations. As Cynthia, the librarian, approaches her, she quickly makes her way out the door.*
>
> *Several days later, Cynthia notices the same woman is back. She does the same thing—walks around the library and exits when Cynthia tries to approach her.*
>
> *A week later she is back. She is looking at some pamphlets displayed on a shelf. Cynthia approaches her with a little smile and says, jovially, "You must like the snow to be out and about today! Some*

snowstorm we had last night, wasn't it?" The woman looks up and says, "Why, yes! We got seven inches of snow at our house! I live just a few blocks away, so I walked over."

Cynthia nods her head and, looking the woman in the eye, says, "Well, you're very brave! You know, I don't think I've seen you in the library before. I just want to make sure you know that every visit to the Health Library is private and our staff keeps all information requests confidential. We understand how important protecting privacy is. It's the law and it's also the right thing to do."

The woman nods her head in agreement.

"So, what brings you to the library today on such a cold, snowy morning?"

"Well," she hesitates and then says softly, "My mom has something called a T-I-A, and I just wonder, what is that? Is it something she can die from?"

Cynthia says, "I can help you learn about TIAs. Where would you like to start? With a brief written description? Or a video clip?"

"I think something written, something that I can take home, would be best," the woman says.

Helpful Policies

Being proactive and having written policies in place to deal with patron behavior problems is highly recommended. A good policy provides the framework you need when negotiating difficult patron encounters and ensures that library patrons will receive a fair and rational approach when problems arise. Two such helpful policies, regarding acceptable behavior and patron complaints, are discussed here.

Acceptable Behavior Policy

Human behavior can be heartwarming or heart-wrenching. It can be engaging or infuriating. You may see a variety of behaviors in a consumer health library—most acceptable, some entirely inappropriate. Your consumer health library may want to consider an acceptable behavior policy. An acceptable behavior policy outlines what conduct in the library is suitable and what conduct is not. It is used to prevent and, if necessary, respond to conduct problems in the library. It defines inappropriate behavior in the library and its consequences. An acceptable behavior policy supports the library's mission and is written in accordance with local, state, and federal laws. If your consumer health library is located within a hospital or sponsoring organization, the larger institutional policy on behavior may apply.

In writing such a policy, you'll want to include:

- the rationale for the policy,

- definitions of inappropriate behavior,

- consequences, and

- a statement of fairness in how the policy is applied.

When writing an acceptable behavior policy, seek legal counsel and review. You may need to enforce the policy and you must be sure it is lawful. Once a draft is finalized, you'll want your governing board to approve it.

What types of unacceptable conduct might you consider including? There's a whole host of possibilities, including but not limited to smoking or using tobacco products, illegal Internet activity, being under the influence of alcohol or illegal drugs, verbally or physically harassing staff or other patrons, or making loud, disruptive noises. For a wonderful example, see Exhibit 6-1, Rules of Conduct—The Seattle Public Library.

Enforcing the Policy

You'll want to post your acceptable behavior policy in a prominent place where users can see it. You want it to be accessible so you are able to point and refer to it, should you need to enforce it. It's very important to train your staff in understanding the policy and how to implement it. Once again, role-playing is paramount

Exhibit 6-1. Rules of Conduct— The Seattle Public Library

Welcome to The Seattle Public Library.

The Library is supported by the taxes of the people of Seattle who expect each of our facilities to be clean, comfortable, and safe places for selecting materials, reading, researching, studying, writing, and attending programs and meetings. To this end, the Library is responsible for establishing rules of conduct to protect the rights and safety of Library patrons, volunteers, and staff, and for preserving and protecting the Library's materials, equipment, facilities, and grounds. In addition, the Library has a strong commitment to intellectual freedom and to freedom of access to information.

Enforcement of these rules will be conducted in a fair and reasonable manner. Library staff and/or Seattle Police Officers will intervene to stop prohibited activities and behaviors. Failure to comply with the Library's established rules, regulations, and policies could result in removal from the premises and exclusion from the Library for a period of one day to one year, or in arrest or prosecution. Violations could also result in the restriction and/or termination of Library privileges, including the use of Library computers and other equipment (RCW 27.12.290).

Individual patrons have the right to request an administrative review of an exclusion order that is for a period greater than seven days (The Seattle Public Library Policy #3j, Rules of Conduct Enforcement).

(Cont'd.)

Exhibit 6-1 *(Continued)*

For the comfort and safety of patrons, volunteers, and staff, and the protection of Library property, the following actions are examples of conduct not allowed on Library property:

- Engaging in any activity in violation of Federal, State, local or other applicable law, or Library policy.
- Failing to comply with a reasonable staff request.
- Carrying firearms and dangerous weapons of any type (except by law enforcement officers and authorized security personnel of The Seattle Public Library).
- Being under the influence of alcohol/illegal drugs, and selling, using, or possessing alcohol/illegal drugs.
- Verbally or physically threatening or harassing other patrons, volunteers, or staff, including stalking, staring, lurking, offensive touching, and obscene acts such as sex acts and indecent exposure.
- Soliciting or conducting surveys not authorized by the Library.
- Stealing, damaging, altering, or inappropriate use of Library property in Library facilities or on Library grounds, including computer hardware and software, printers (The Seattle Public Library Policy #6g, Public Use of the Internet), copiers, phones, and other equipment.
- Trespassing in nonpublic areas, being in the Library without permission of an authorized Library employee before or after Library operating hours, or camping on Library grounds.
- Fighting or challenging to fight, running, pushing, shoving, or throwing things.

(Cont'd.)

Exhibit 6-1 *(Continued)*

- Creating disruptive noises such as loud talking, screaming, or banging on computer keyboards.
- Gambling and group activities which are disruptive to the Library environment.
- Using audible devices without headphones or with headphones set at a volume that disturbs others. Using cell phones, pagers, and other communication devices in a manner that disturbs others. Audible cell phone and pager ringers must be turned off.
- Using restrooms for bathing or shampooing, doing laundry, or changing clothes.
- Littering.
- Smoking, chewing, and other tobacco use on Library property.
- Entering or being in the Library barefoot, without a shirt, with offensive body odor or personal hygiene, or being otherwise attired so as to be disruptive to the Library environment.
- Consuming food or beverages in public areas of the Library not authorized by the Library Food and Beverage Guidelines (The Seattle Public Library Administrative Procedure 070-APP-805, Food and Beverage Rule Guidelines).
- Bringing in articles that measure more than 14"W x 17"H x 20"D.
- Leaving packages, backpacks, luggage, or any other personal items unattended. These unattended items are subject to immediate confiscation.
- Using wheeled devices in Library property or on Library grounds, except in designated areas, including use of skateboards, roller-skates, bicycles, motorized or non-motorized scooters, and shopping carts (except for motorized ADA assistive devices, wheelchairs, walkers, and strollers).

(Cont'd.)

Exhibit 6-1 *(Continued)*

- Moving Library furniture from where it is placed by Library staff. Lying down or sleeping in the restrooms, or on any floor, or couch, table or seat in the Library; having feet on furniture; or blocking aisles, exits or entrances.
- Neglecting to provide proper supervision of children (The Seattle Public Library Policy #6h, Unattended Children).
- Bringing pets or animals, other than service animals necessary for disabilities, into the Library, except as authorized by the City Librarian.

Individuals with disabilities may request reasonable accommodation by calling (206) 386-4110 or emailing administrative.review@spl.org.

DATE ADOPTED: April 27, 2006
DATE EFFECTIVE: July 10, 2006
SUPERCEDES POLICY: Rules of Conduct Policy adopted May 27, 1997, and revised January 22, 2002, and March 16, 2004. Used with permission.

in teaching your staff enforcement skills. They need practice and experience before they can be expected to have a difficult conversation with an unruly patron. It takes confidence to approach someone and ask him or her to comply with your policy on acceptable behavior; confidence can be built through practice. In your training efforts, teach your staff to document their enforcement efforts. This paperwork is critical if further incidents occur or if enforcement is challenged by a patron.

When you encounter a violation of your acceptable behavior policy, first analyze the situation. Use the four-step approach: stop, breathe, reflect, and choose. After calming yourself and gaining clarity regarding the situation, decide, how serious is this?

If you need to proceed, respond by using a matter-of-fact tone of voice. Be calm and nonthreatening, but firm. State that the *behavior*, not the individual, is "inappropriate" or "unacceptable." Refer to the posted policy being violated. Do not argue with the patron; just restate the facts in the same calm, nonthreatening voice. Use your knowledge of handling angry patrons here. Give the individual a choice, if possible, in how to resolve the unacceptable behavior.

If you can, have other staff members with you when you enforce the policy. In using additional staff, your body language as a group is important here. Instead of lining your staff up like a football team on the 50-yard line directly across from the patron, have your staff stand behind you in a reverse V-formation, the same pattern geese use when flying. The first stance is very confrontational and tells the patron, "We're ganging up on you." The second stance is much softer and indicates to the patron, "I have all these people behind me and supporting me."

Always take the threat of violence seriously. If possible, never block entrances or exits when enforcing an acceptable behavior policy. Call 911 or security if things get out of hand. Again, make sure you document the incident. Exhibit 6-2 shows a sample Unacceptable Behavior Incident Report form.

Establishing clear expectations regarding acceptable behavior through the development and implementation of a policy can help prevent behavior problems from occurring in the consumer health library. Having an acceptable behavior policy also provides the necessary enforcement tool should unacceptable behavior occur. Although this is the worst-case scenario, it is better to be prepared. Let this be your motto: Prepare for the worst, and hope for the best!

> *Denise is working in the consumer health library and she sees a patron reading the newspaper and talking loudly, at times swearing to himself. Other users nearby are giving worried looks. Some are rolling their eyes and others are moving away.*

Denise knows she must enforce the library's acceptable behavior policy. She asks her two co-workers, Laurel and Meredith, to accompany her. The three approach the patron, with Laurel and Meredith flanking Denise and standing slightly behind her, like geese.

"Excuse me, sir," Denise states. "You may not be aware, but you are shouting and swearing and that behavior is in violation of the library's acceptable behavior policy. I need to ask your cooperation. You may calm down or you must leave."

The patron looks at Denise and the co-workers behind her. "What?!" he shouts. "I was not! I was simply enjoying the newspaper. Geez! Give me a break!" he thunders.

Denise calmly restates, "Sir, you are shouting and swearing and that behavior is in violation of the library's acceptable behavior policy. I would greatly appreciate your assistance. You may calm down or you must leave."

The man scowls, "Well, since I'm not finished yet, I will try to be more quiet."

Denise and her co-workers return to their duties. The man's behavior is appropriate for the duration of his library visit. Denise documents the incident and gives the paperwork to the library director.

Policies for Handling Complaints

Handling patron complaints was discussed earlier in this chapter and establishing appropriate policies for this purpose is both pro-active and ensures fairness in resolving complaints. Exhibit 6-3 provides an example of a policy for handling complaints regarding objectionable library materials.

Exhibit 6-2. Unacceptable Behavior Incident Report

Today's date: _____

Staff member's name: _____

Date and time of incident: _____

Name and description of individual involved:

_____

_____

Describe the incident: _____

_____

_____

Names of witnesses: _____

_____

How was the incident resolved? _____

_____

_____

_____

Signature of staff member/Date

Exhibit 6-3. Patron Complaint Policy Regarding Objectionable Materials

I. Purpose

The purpose of this policy is to provide a method for patrons to submit complaints to the _____ Library regarding objectionable material.

II. Policy

1. A patron with a complaint about objectionable library material must submit objections in writing to the library director.

2. The library director will review the complaint to make sure that it pertains to material actually owned by the library.

3. If it is a valid complaint, a copy of the written complaint will be sent to the library's administrative director.

4. The library director will investigate the complaint using the Collection Development Policy as an evaluation tool. A benchmark of reputable book reviews and other information sources will be researched. The library director will issue a written report of findings. A copy of the report will be sent to the library's administrative director.

5. Together, the library director and the administrative director will make a presentation to the_____Hospital Board. The Board will determine the appropriateness of the material at its next meeting. The Board's decision regarding the material is final.

6. A written response regarding the complaint's resolution will be mailed to the patron by the_____Hospital Board secretary.

Summary

As a consumer health librarian, you will witness the best and the worst of human behavior. By using the appropriate verbal and nonverbal communication skills outlined in this chapter, you can manage a range of difficult patrons—from the angry person to the complainer to the frequent flyer to the guarded individual. In stressful encounters, remember to practice the four-step approach: stop, breathe, reflect, and *choose* how to respond. These four steps will help to calm you, ground you, and give you the clarity you need to deal with a trying situation. Most difficult patrons are in some type of emotional pain and will respond to calmness and reason. Time and experience will help you hone these skills.

While you can't prescribe patron conduct, you can have policies in place for responding to a variety of patron behaviors. Acceptable behavior policies are best written *before* there is a problem, and they should be displayed in a prominent place. Practicing enforcement through role-playing at staff meetings helps to reinforce the skills needed to respond appropriately in stressful encounters. Policies should also be in place for patrons to lodge complaints. Sound policies coupled with solid communication skills are essential ingredients for successful librarian-patron interaction in the consumer health library.

Reference

Benson, Herbert, and Eileen M. Stuart. 1992. *The Wellness Book: The Comprehensive Guide to Maintaining Health and Treating Stress-related Illness*. New York: Fireside.

Chapter 7

Self-care for the Health Information Provider

In a nutshell, consumer health reference work is stressful. On a typical day, a consumer health librarian is likely to encounter patron questions such as the following:

- "My mom has metastatic breast cancer. Would you have any information on pain control? The doctors have tried just about everything. Now they want to put her on methadone. Isn't that used by drug addicts?"

- "My son is having violent seizures. He's three years old. They've done a million tests and now the doctor said something about Lennox-Gastaut syndrome? He tried to tell me what it was, but I just didn't understand. Something about mental retardation? How can this be—we're talking about my baby!"

- "My daughter is in end-stage renal failure and is undergoing treatment in a hospital 1,200 miles away. Her husband tells us it doesn't look good. I need to go and be with her but I just don't have the means. Is there any financial assistance available for me to be able to fly back there and be with her?"

Dealing with such difficult reference questions, where the answers might seriously impact someone's life, may take its toll on your health if you don't take care of yourself. While the goal is to practice consumer health librarianship with compassionate neutrality, the truth is, the rigors of our work do seep in. Somewhere in our consciousness we take it to heart. Failing to deal effectively with the emotional pressures that we are exposed to each day can affect our overall health and well-being.

That said, the larger truth is, *all* jobs are stressful. Given our country's Puritan work ethic, we accept stress as part of the price we must pay for gainful employment and, in fact, we tend to glamorize it. Think about the conversations you have with coworkers; the phrase "I'm so stressed out!" is heard so often it's become meaningless. We wear our stress as a badge of honor, when in fact there is a causal relationship between high levels of stress and heart disease, the number-one killer in the United States (Ramachandruni, Handberg, and Sheps, 2004). This is nothing to gloat about.

Health Effects of Stress

We're so overly familiar with stress that we don't take it seriously. Perhaps if we better understood it, we'd see the importance of doing our best to manage it.

Stress comes in two different forms: good stress and bad stress. The good stress is the kind that energizes us—makes us feel vibrant and alive and ready to take on the world. Scientists call this "eustress." The bad stress is the kind most of us think of when we use the word "stress" around the watercooler to anyone who will listen. It's the stress that makes us tired, changes our mood, and makes us feel "out of control." Scientists call this "distress." In this chapter, when we talk about stress, we are referring to *distress*.

So just what is stress? Stress may be defined as the inability to cope with and manage the competing demands in our lives. When we're stressed, the demands have the upper hand—we feel overwhelmed, burdened, fatigued.

Although nature has beautifully equipped our body with the ability to respond to a threat or a stress, we unnecessarily push this innate mechanism to the limit in today's world. This inborn ability to handle a stressor is known as the fight-or-flight response. Because it is automatic, we don't have to consciously think about preparing our body to respond. And our body's response is nothing short of phenomenal.

Say it's 50,000 years ago and you are out hunting and gathering, when you see a saber-toothed tiger staring directly at you. You would perceive this as a stressful situation—a threat. In such a situation, your body would automatically respond by:

- increasing your metabolism;

- upping your heart rate, blood pressure, breathing rate, and cholesterol;

- tensing your muscles;

- releasing additional glucose into your bloodstream;

- affecting your digestive system, resulting in difficulty swallowing, dry mouth, and diarrhea or constipation; and

- releasing powerful hormones, such as cortisol (also known as "the stress hormone"), into your bloodstream (Benson, 1975).

These physiological changes help protect us from harm. They prepare our body to either physically fight a threat or, conversely, flee it. As we successfully fight or flee, we dissipate the physiological energy we have activated and return our body to its normal state of well-being.

The days where most humans have to fight off tigers for their physical survival are long gone. However, the fight-or-flight response lives on, and for good reason. Say, for example, we work in a busy city and step off a curb as a car is careening around the corner. Immediately our fight-or-flight response is engaged—an appropriate physical response to a life-threatening situation. As we move out of the path of the oncoming car, we dissipate the physiological changes in our body, returning it to its normal state.

This is all well and good. However, in today's world, most stress is not to our physical safety, as in the previous example, but is *psychological* in origin—work, family, money, relationships, and the like. Yet our body still responds to psychological stress with the same fight-or-flight response. After all, a perceived threat—be it to our emotional or our physical health—is still a threat. Our body doesn't distinguish between the two.

Every time our body senses a stressful situation, the fight-or-flight response kicks in, changing our body chemistry. These repeated instinctive chemical changes are not good for our overall health and well-being. A fight-or-flight response that is constantly "on" over time will lead to chronic, unhealthy physiology, and eventually to serious health problems. It doesn't take a Noble Prize–winning physician to see that if our blood pressure is chronically elevated due to stress, we may someday have a stroke or heart attack. Similarly, chronically elevated cholesterol levels may lead to heart disease, elevated blood glucose may lead to diabetes, and so on.

Fortunately, much of how we respond to psychological stress is within our control. Our attitudes, beliefs, and thoughts have a lot to do with how our body recognizes and responds to daily stresses. How we understand a situation and choose to respond will determine whether the fight-or-flight response kicks in automatically or we are able to interrupt it and drain its harmful chemical bath. To interrupt the automatic stress response requires great self-awareness and the use of effective coping skills. We're so used to minimizing stress in our culture that we don't recognize its deleterious effect on our body, mind, or spirit. Many of us function on autopilot. We go through our day without a lot of conscious thought about how we are feeling or coping; we just know we are stressed. So, how *do* we recognize stress? How do we *identify* it? *Name* it? Using a simple stress self-awareness tool such as the Stress Mapper (Exhibit 7-1) may help.

To use this tool, simply sit down and think hard about the past week. As you recall it, ask yourself, "Which, if any, of the symptoms listed on the Stress Mapper did I notice or experience?" Check *all* those that apply. Now each week for one month, return

Exhibit 7-1. Stress Mapper

Symptom	Week 1	Week 2	Week 3	Week 4
Back pain				
Bored or listless				
Bouts of crying				
Canker sore				
Cranky; testy with others				
Eating too much				
Feeling extra tired				
Feeling isolated				
Feeling like you've lost direction or have no direction				
Feeling overwhelmed				
Feeling restless				
Forgetfulness				
Grinding teeth during sleep				
Headache				
Heart palpitations				
Humorless				
Inability to make simple decisions				
Loss of creativity or creative drive				
Lowered sex drive or lack of intimacy				
Muscle tightness (neck & shoulders)				
Nagging				
Nail biting				
Nervousness or anxiety				
No appetite				
On edge; easy to anger or criticize				
Resuming or increased cigarette smoking				
Too much alcohol				
Trouble concentrating; brain fog				
Trouble sleeping				
Trouble with memory/ remembering				
Upset stomach				
Withdrawing from loved ones, friends, coworkers				

to the Stress Mapper tool and ask yourself the same question, "Which, if any, of the symptoms listed did I have?" Continue to check all that apply.

At the end of one month, review the entire tool. Are there symptoms you have checked every time? Symptoms you've checked two or three times? You will probably notice a series of check marks after certain symptoms. These are your self-awareness clues indicating when you are stressed.

For example, I often thought I was just having a bad morning on those days when I couldn't find my car keys. I didn't pay attention to this as a symptom of stress until I did the Stress Mapper tool. I consider myself to be a highly organized individual (aren't all librarians?) and I assumed when I couldn't locate my car keys, which I typically keep in the same place when I am home, that it was just bad luck. After using the Stress Mapper tool, I realized my occasional "forgetfulness" was a symptom of too much stress. Now on mornings when I can't find my car keys, I recognize that I have too much on my to-do list. Forgetfulness is one of my symptoms of too much stress. In order to take care of myself, I take simple steps to address the stress in my life, rather than ignoring it and hoping it will just go away.

At the end of the month, you, too, will have a list of clues that will inform you when your stress plate is too full. Your self-awareness will alert you to the need to take action to lessen the stress in your life. Once you respond to stress, you regain a measure of control over your life and you diminish its harmful effects. By definition, stress makes us feel unable to cope with or manage the demands of our life; we feel out of control. By recognizing the symptoms of stress and acting to relieve them, you regain control. You cannot respond to something you are unaware of, so self-study is crucial. In some circles this is known as "living in awareness."

Once you recognize a symptom of stress, it's important to identify its source. The physical symptoms you identify are warning lights, advising you to look more deeply into what is causing your stress. Suppose your neck aches and you're aware that this is a stress warning signal. Ask yourself, "What's really going on?"

Too many long days spent at the reference desk with countless demanding or emotionally taxing patrons? You're late with your car payment and fretting about a possible penalty, so it's hard to concentrate at work? It's important to be clear where the stress is coming from in order to respond to it effectively.

Here's the central question to ask yourself: "Is the source of my stress something I can change or affect?" If the answer is "yes," then the best thing you can do is to problem-solve it. Think about the situation and identify potential solutions, listing both merits and disadvantages of each; seek the wisdom of others whose opinions you respect; reflect on your options; and then choose one solution that you feel is best. Finally, pick a time to implement your solution and *follow through* with it. The act of problem solving reduces stress by giving you back your sense of power and control over a situation you thought was out of your control. When you stop, think, and work things through, you interrupt the stress response.

Linda's been working the reference desk every day for weeks. Her shifts are long and lately she's noticed her shoulders begin to ache after arriving at work. It seems as if every person she helps is very needy. Today she's helped:

- *A woman with stage IV breast cancer find end-of-life information; the woman shared her regrets that she won't see her children grow up.*

- *A teen wanting to know where he can get an HIV test without his parents' knowledge; he's gay and if his parents find out they'll kill him.*

- *An elderly gentlemen who is losing his wife to Alzheimer's and needs to consider getting outside help; he reminisces about their life together and begins to cry softly, and on and on.*

That evening when Linda returns home, she pulls out a Stress Mapper that one of her coworkers shared. She filled it out for a month and she now knows that "tight neck, shoulders" is a sign of stress for her. Of course it would be; she has the weight of the world on her shoulders! She asks herself, "What's stressing me? Work? Things at home?" After mulling this over for a while she is certain it is those long days at the reference desk that have been feeling very heavy. "Is this something I might be able to change?" she wonders. She decides it's worth trying. So after dinner she sits down and writes out a list of possible solutions:

1. Quit!

2. Ask my supervisor for shorter shifts.

3. Call in sick!

After looking at the pluses and minuses for each possible solution, Linda decides to focus on #2—asking for shorter shifts at the reference desk. Perhaps instead of the one long four-hour block at the reference desk, she can ask to be scheduled for two two-hour blocks spread throughout the workday. The next day she approaches her supervisor and has a respectful conversation about reference desk scheduling. Her supervisor says, "I thought our staff would prefer getting their reference desk shifts over all at once. I guess I was wrong! I can put you on shorter shifts with next week's schedule. Will that be soon enough for you?" Linda is happy and notices her shoulders already feel lighter than air.

In some situations, you can't exert a measure of control or effect change. Sometimes, for reasons beyond our control, we must simply bear a stressful situation. Say, for example, you are a solo librarian and must field reference questions all day, every day. Perhaps you've asked for more staff and have been denied. You're actively looking for another position, but in the meantime, you must be employed. In this case, you are in a situation you must bear and it's important to practice stress reduction techniques through good self-care in order to minimize the damage to your health.

Self-care includes many things, one of which is a physical approach, such as using physical exercise or activity to relieve stress. It could be a walk, a bike ride, yoga, karate, dancing, bowling—anything that gets you active and allows your body to rid itself of the muscle and mental fatigue brought on by the stress response. The literature is full of reports on the health benefits of exercise and it is a perfect antidote to stress. Other physical antidotes include taking a hot bath, getting a massage, laughing (for example, watching a comedy DVD or reading a funny book), and participating in a hobby—gardening, knitting, cross-stitching, kite-flying—whatever strikes your fancy and physically engages you.

Self-care also means choosing activities to relieve emotional distress. Journaling thoughts and feelings, practicing acceptance, seeking the support of others, using positive self-talk (seeing the glass half-full instead of half-empty), and even a good cry all help dissipate stress.

Let's revisit Linda's situation. Suppose that this time her supervisor has a different response.

> *"Linda, we've lost one staff member and the other is on vacation. I'm right in the middle of departmental budgeting for next year and reviewing applicants for the open position. I'm sorry, but you'll just have to step up and continue to staff the desk this way until Ray returns from vacation, and then we'll see what we can do. I'm sorry."*
>
> *Linda is not happy. She knows now that she must bear the situation; her shoulders still ache and she is tired. She remembers the handout her coworker shared with her. It said something about "When you can't change a situation, get physically active to reduce stress." She goes home and decides to try a new yoga class at the "Y" down the street. What can it hurt? She throws on some old sweatpants and a T-shirt and heads to the class.*
>
> *The instructor asks, "Anyone have a special part of the body they'd like to work tonight?"*

> *Linda sheepishly raises her hand and says, "Well,*
> *my shoulders are really tight." "No problem—we can*
> *gently stretch them. Just be sure not to do any stretch*
> *to the point of pain. Now let's begin." After class,*
> *Linda feels wonderful—no more aching shoulders*
> *and work seems a million miles away.*

Self-care for less stress is often difficult for women, and librarianship is a profession that is predominantly female. Women are socialized to be caretakers and often end up at the very bottom of their own to-do list. This is particularly true of boomers and those beyond—another proportionately larger segment of the library profession. As the flight attendants remind us every time we fly, "In case of loss of cabin pressure, an oxygen mask will fall from the overhead compartment. Please *first put on your own oxygen mask before assisting others in your care.*" These simple instructions serve as a stark reminder that if we don't tend to our own needs, particularly when times are tough, we won't be much good to anyone else. Tending to our need for stress reduction can't wait. The health effects of stress are too detrimental. As women, we can make our health and self-care a higher priority. It isn't being selfish, as many of us have been socialized to believe. It's vital, like putting our own oxygen mask on first, so we are alive and able to care for others in our life.

The 24/7 Stress Antidote

Sometimes you need immediate relief from stress. The good news is that you carry it with you always; it's just a breath away. You can guide your breath at any time to help relieve stress. Herbert Benson coined the term "the relaxation response" after he studied the use of meditation or focused breath work to lower blood pressure. He discovered that this technique brought about a complete reversal of the physiological effects of the fight-or-flight response (Benson, 1975).

To use your breath as an antidote to stress, you need to set the stage. Ideally, you want a quiet space. It doesn't have to be big, just a place where you will not be distracted by noise or other people. To begin, sit comfortably in a chair with both feet on the floor, your arms relaxed at your sides. Or lie down on your bed or on the floor. As you settle in, choose a word, a phrase, an image, or even a prayer that is comforting to you; you will use this in the exercise. Now, close your eyes and take a deep breath in through your nose—a belly breath—one that makes your abdomen pooch out. Then, exhale. Try to make the length of your in-breath the same as that of your out-breath. You may want to count: 1-2-3-4-5 as you inhale, 1-2-3-4-5 as you exhale. Repeat this step two more times, until you have taken three deep breaths. Now relax and release into the natural rhythm of your breathing. No worries, just let it flow.

Remember the comforting word, phrase, image, or prayer that you chose at the beginning of this exercise? Say it to yourself as you relax and release into the natural rhythm of your breath. I like to use the word "calm" on the in-breath and the word "relaxed" on the out-breath. As I do this exercise I find that as I breathe in, I become calm, and as I breathe out, I become relaxed. By the end of a short breathing session, *I am calm and relaxed.*

If your mind wanders and distracting thoughts creep in—your to-do list, the conversation you had with your spouse this morning, the new software you'll be testing at work—just release them. These distracting thoughts are normal and bound to occur. Our minds are busy and not used to being still or quiet. In fact, in Buddhism, the racing mind is called "monkey mind" because our thoughts are analogous to monkeys in the rain forest playfully leaping from tree to tree. When your mind wanders or leaps from tree to tree, just gently pull it back to your focus word, phrase, or image. If you are prone to imagery, you might imagine your monkey-mind thoughts as helium balloons, and gently let them go as they occur. You can watch them drift skyward as you concentrate on your focus word.

Using your breath to literally slow life down reverses the ill effects of the fight-or-flight response. As you experience Benson's relaxation response, you will calm both your body and your mind. For health benefits, use this technique 20 minutes each day. As you use your breath as a stress-reduction tool, you will find that you remain calmer in stressful situations; have greater clarity of thought, enabling you to better focus on your work and your life in general; and feel more energetic. This magnificent tool is something that is within your control, always available to you, and affordable.

As you learn to use your breath for relaxation, you'll find that this technique comes in handy for many occasions when you need to calm down and quickly regroup—for example, before answering a difficult telephone call, when helping a demanding patron, or when your computer is running so slowly that you wonder why you should use it at all. A deep breath in through your nose and correspondingly lengthy breath out will help restore your inner peace.

Stress Buffers

Research by Suzanne Kobasa and associates suggests that there are certain personal characteristics that protect individuals from stress. She studied individuals who did not succumb to health problems although they were under a great deal of stress and found that they share similar attitudes, beliefs, and behaviors. She called these attributes "stress hardiness," meaning such people were less vulnerable to the effects of stress, and described the attributes as commitment, control, and challenge (Kobasa, 1979). Today, a body of evidence has emerged to include a fourth one: connection (DeLongis and Holtzman, 2005).

Individuals who are committed to their work, a cause, or a mission and believe that what they are doing is meaningful and matters are better able to cope with the stresses of life.

Control refers to individuals who believe that they have control over their life—they live in conscious awareness that their choices and actions make a difference. They are the captain of their ship, so to speak, and feel that they set the sail and direct the course of their own life.

The attribute of challenge describes those individuals who think positively—these people are optimistic. They see a problem not as a threat, but as an opportunity to learn something new in order to master it. They are challenged by life and enjoy rising to the challenge.

Finally, connection refers to individuals who have strong relationships and the support of loved ones—family, friends, coworkers, and so on. It also includes those individuals who have an active faith or spiritual life—a connection to something deeper and everlasting.

Stress hardiness characteristics serve as a buffer against stress. Do you have these attributes? If not, you may want to develop them in your life to help shield you from the ill effects of chronic stress. Use the 4-Cs for Reducing Stress Worksheet (Exhibit 7-2) to help you identify your stress hardiness.

Support for Self-care

Sometimes, try as you might to employ effective coping mechanisms, you find you just can't manage. Your stress feels constant and overwhelming. Other indications that you are having trouble coping are: poor sleep, rapid gain or loss of weight, obsessive thoughts about your problem(s), withdrawal from your friends and family, and frequent, irrational emotional outbursts. This is the time to seek outside professional support—help from a licensed mental health therapist. There is no need to tough it out; you just need a little help putting on your oxygen mask. Your employee health plan may help with reimbursement for visits to licensed mental health therapists, such as a licensed clinical social worker, clinical psychologist, or psychiatrist. Ask your doctor or primary care provider for a recommendation.

When you make your first appointment, confirm that the therapist has experience in treating people with problems such as yours and then ask what kind of therapy is provided, how much it costs, and whether or not your insurance is accepted. Knowing what to expect before the first visit may relieve your anxiety about going. Seeking professional support when necessary is an important tool in your self-care toolkit and may be just the ticket you need to start feeling better.

Exhibit 7-2. 4-Cs for Reducing Stress Worksheet

Stress-hardy people share four common characteristics: Control, Commitment, Challenge, and Connection. Use this worksheet to address the four Cs in your life.

Control/Influence

Individuals who embrace ownership of their work and feel that their choices influence or impact their work manage to have better overall health.

I feel ownership of my work and I set the direction of my work by:

1. _____
2. _____
3. _____

Commitment

Individuals who are committed to the mission of their work, believe that their work has meaning, and have a take-charge attitude toward their work often experience less stress.

I commit to my own self-care in the workplace or take charge of my work by:

1. _____
2. _____
3. _____

(Cont'd.)

Exhibit 7-2 *(Continued)*

Challenge

Individuals who have a positive attitude and who feel that they can learn and master new job skills or job demands are better able to cope.

Three things I can do to learn new job skills or to meet my job demands are:

1. _____

2. _____

3. _____

Closeness/Connection

Individuals who have support from loved ones, friends, or co-workers generally experience less stress. Less stress means better health overall.

Individuals or groups I feel close or connected to and who will support me in my work are:

1. _____

2. _____

3. _____

Summary

As a health librarian, you have a number of tools at your disposal to conquer stress: self-awareness, problem solving, physical and emotional coping techniques, meditation or breath work, and developing and relying upon stress-hardiness characteristics. Employing these tools will help you cope with your job demands and practice your reference work with compassionate neutrality. More important, it is crucial for your well-being to take stress seriously so it does not take its toll on your *health*. Perhaps you will be the one to move the watercooler conversation from "I'm so stressed out!" to "I'm coping well with the stress of my life and really living each day—aren't you?"

Additional Reading

Wood, Jeffrey C., and Matthew McKay. 2007. *Getting Help: The Complete & Authoritative Guide to Self-Assessment & Treatment of Mental Health Problems*. Oakland, CA: New Harbinger.

References

Benson, Herbert. 1975. *The Relaxation Response*. New York: Avon Books.

DeLongis, Anita, and Susan Holtzman. 2005. "Coping in Context: The Role of Stress, Social Support, and Personality in Coping." *Journal of Personality* 73, no. 6 (December): 1633–1656.

Kobasa, S. 1979. "Stressful Life Events, Personality, and Health: An Inquiry into Hardiness." *Journal of Personality and Social Psychology* 37, no. 1 (January): 1–11.

Ramachandruni, S., E. Handberg, and D. S. Sheps. 2004. "Acute and Chronic Psychological Stress in Coronary Disease." *Current Opinion in Cardiology* 19, no. 5 (September): 494–499.

Index

Page numbers followed by the letter "f" indicate figures.

Q

Quick Tips—When Talking with Your Doctor, 11

R

Radiation therapy, 29
Rainie, Lee, 9
Ramachandrundi, S., 116
Rapid cycling, 33–34
Reading material about an illegal activity, 39–40
Reference. *See also* Patrons
  body language, 19–21, 92, 102
  confidential inquiries, 23, 43–45
  eye contact, 20, 93, 102–103
  friendliness, 79–80
  interview techniques, 27–29
  open-ended questions, 102
  self-control, 90–91
  setting up, 23
  skills, keeping up-to-date, 64
  special reference interview tips, 26f
  symptoms of stress, 119–122
"Reference Etiquette: A Guide to Excruciatingly Correct Behavior" (Eckwright, Hoskisson, and Pollastro), 36
"The Reference Interview Revisited: Librarian-Patron Interaction in the Virtual Environment" (Curry), 36
Referrals, 64
Reflect, and Four-Step Approach, 90
Refugee Health Information Network (RHIN), 81
Religious conflicts, 38–40
Renal failure, 115
Repeated questions by patron, 98–101
Respect, 51
Responsibility, return of, 99
Rights, library, 11, 52, 57
Rules of Conduct, 106f–109f

Rx Assist Patient Assistance Program Center, 71
Rx Outreach, 71

S

Safe sex, 83
Safeguards for professional practice, 58, 59f-60f
Sample disclaimer, 59f–60f
Scacco, Linda, 75
Schizophrenia, 46, 73f
Scope of practice, 54
Seattle/King County LGBT Health Web Pages, 84f
Seattle Public Library, Rules of Conduct, 106f-109f
Seborrheic dermatitis, 8–9
Security, 93
Seizures, 115
Selected Patient Information Resources in Asian Languages (Spiral), 81f
Self-awareness and communication guidelines and strategies, 21–23, 49
Self-care for health information provider
  fight-or-flight response, 117–118, 124
  health effects of stress, 115–118, 120–124
  self-care support, 127
  stress buffers, 126–127
  stress mapper, 118, 119f, 120–121
  24/7 stress antidote, 124–126
  worksheet for reducing stress, 128f–129f
Self-control, 90–91
Self-diagnosis, 61
Service, level of, 50
Sheps, D. S., 116
Sielski, Lester M., 36
Skills, keeping up-to-date, 64
Skin cancer, 82
Smith, David M., 83

About the Author

A writer, teacher, and consultant, **Michele Spatz** is past president of the Oregon Health Sciences Libraries Association and former chair of the Consumer and Patient Health Information Section of the Medical Library Association; she has taught two MLA CE courses on consumer health information over the past ten years. An alumnus of the University of Illinois, Urbana, she earned her BS as a park naturalist, and her master's degree in Library and Information Science. As branch library director at the University of Illinois College of Medicine in Peoria, Michele was the campus's first librarian to earn tenure. In 1991, she moved to The Dalles, Oregon, to establish the Planetree Health Resource Center, a community-based consumer health library, for Mid-Columbia Medical Center. She continues to serve as its director.